Emergency Medicine Case-Based Guide

Adeola A. Kosoko

Editor

Emergency Medicine Case-Based Guide

Obstetric Emergencies

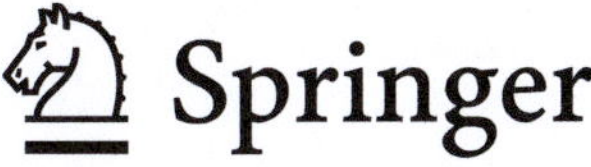

Editor
Adeola A. Kosoko
Department of Emergency Medicine
The University of Texas Health Sciences
Center at Houston
Houston, TX, USA

ISBN 978-3-031-70120-7   ISBN 978-3-031-70118-4   (eBook)
https://doi.org/10.1007/978-3-031-70118-4

This Springer imprint is published by the registered company Springer Nature Switzerland AG
The registered company address is: Gewerbestrasse 11, 6330 Cham, Switzerland

If disposing of this product, please recycle the paper.

Preface

Case studies are a great instructive way for clinicians to prepare for their own similar encounters with some familiarity based on someone else's experiences. Each case describes the background of a patient and clues needed to make an appropriate diagnosis. As some of the preeminent diagnosticians in the house of medicine, it is especially important for those practicing in the emergency setting to properly identify potentially life-threatening emergencies in a timely fashion.

This book contains contributions from skilled physicians specially trained in emergency medicine and/or pediatric medicine. It is structured into three major sections: early pregnancy emergencies, late pregnancy emergencies, and neonatal emergencies. Each chapter presents a true-to-life case based on expert experiences. These are the experiences of my esteemed colleagues around the United States of America (USA). These experiences will help give depth to the various ways "can't miss" diagnoses are made and how they can be best managed. These authors have also provided tips and tricks to help uncover a diagnosis and to manage an obstetric emergency even with limited resources.

There are approximately 700 women who die annually in the USA due to pregnancy or its complications. These deaths include during gestation, during labor and delivery, and within the first year postpartum. Furthermore, there are well-documented racial disparities (particularly affecting Black, American Indian, and Alaska Native women) which have persisted for decades affecting maternal and infant health despite numerous advances in medical care. Fortunately, about 80% of pregnancy-related deaths are preventable.

Many obstetric emergencies are rare in their presentation frequency to the emergency department. Though in many situations, obstetric emergencies are directly managed by obstetricians and gynecologists. This book is meant for people who are not obstetricians or gynecologists; people who have a different cognitive skillset and different set of resources. Emergency physicians have a role to play in decreasing the disparities associated with obstetric outcomes and they can improve the outcomes of mothers and babies in the USA. My hope is that this book edifies and empowers emergency physicians in their care of this potentially vulnerable patient population.

My humblest thanks to my collaborators. I am very proud to have completed this labor of love. I am looking forward to doing this again soon!

Houston, TX, USA   Adeola A. Kosoko

Contents

Editor and Contributors

About the Editor

Adeola A. Kosoko is a practicing emergency physician certified by the American Board of Emergency Medicine in both emergency medicine and pediatric emergency medicine. She currently clinically treats "big kids" and "little adults" ages 0 to 110 years in Houston, Texas and especially finds joy in medical education.

She lectures regularly at the McGovern Medical School and the Cizik School of Nursing at the University of Texas Health Sciences Center in Houston, Texas and has published multiple research articles on the topics of medical simulation, optimizing pediatric emergency care, obstetric emergencies, diversity, inclusion, equity, and collaboration in global health. She has also been an invited lecturer for multiple regional, national, and international events, known for her practical and engaging teaching style. She has been hosted by the American College of Emergency Physicians, the American Academy of Emergency Medicine, and the Belize Medical and Dental Association.

Dr. Kosoko has completed post-graduate fellowship training in global health. She spends time researching and working in partnership with international colleagues having developed curricula teaching pediatric emergency medical care to providers in Botswana and Belize.

Contributors

Peter Acker, MD, MPH Department of Emergency Medicine, Stanford University School of Medicine, Stanford, CA, USA

Adedoyin Adesina, MD, MEd Department of Emergency Medicine, Baylor College of Medicine, Houston, TX, USA

Cindy Amilcar, MD Department of Emergency Medicine, McGovern School of Medicine, University of Texas Health Sciences Center at Houston, Houston, TX, USA

Carrie Bakunas, MD Department of Emergency Medicine, McGovern School of Medicine, University of Texas Health Sciences Center at Houston, Houston, TX, USA

Rachel C. Bower, MD Department of Emergency Medicine, McGovern School of Medicine, University of Texas Health Sciences Center at Houston, Houston, TX, USA

Cassandra Bradby, MD Department of Emergency Medicine, East Carolina University Brody School of Medicine, Greenville, NC, USA

Ciaura Brown, MD, MBA Department of Emergency Medicine, Baylor College of Medicine, Houston, TX, USA

Carolina Camacho Ruiz, MD Department of Emergency Medicine, State University of New York Downstate Health Sciences University/King's County Hospital, Brooklyn, NY, USA

Omoyeni O. Clement, MD Department of Emergency Medicine, McGovern School of Medicine, University of Texas Health Sciences Center at Houston, Houston, TX, USA

Suchismita Datta, MD Department of Emergency Medicine, New York University Grossman Long Island School of Medicine, Mineola, NY, USA

Omoefe Ebhohimen, MD Department of Emergency Medicine, State University of New York Downstate Health Sciences University, Brooklyn, NY, USA

Zoë R. Fisher, MD Department of Emergency Medicine, McGovern School of Medicine, University of Texas Health Sciences Center at Houston, Houston, TX, USA

Sadia Jamshad, MD Department of Emergency Medicine, McGovern School of Medicine, University of Texas Health Sciences Center at Houston, Houston, TX, USA

Juliana Jaramillo, MD Department of Emergency Medicine, East Carolina University Brody School of Medicine, Greenville, NC, USA

Jodi D. Jones, MD Department of Emergency Medicine, University of Texas Southwestern Medical Center, Dallas, TX, USA

Adeola A. Kosoko, MD Department of Emergency Medicine, McGovern School of Medicine, University of Texas Health Sciences Center at Houston, Houston, TX, USA

Carolina Mendoza, MD, MBA Department of Emergency Medicine, University of Maryland School of Medicine, Baltimore, MD, USA

Asha Morrow, MD Department of Pediatrics, Baylor College of Medicine/Texas Children's Hospital, Houston, TX, USA

Monalisa Muchatuta, MD, MS Department of Emergency Medicine, State University of New York Downstate Health Sciences University, Brooklyn, NY, USA

Marquita S. Norman, MD, MBA Department of Emergency Medicine, University of Texas Southwestern Medical Center, Dallas, TX, USA

Felisha Perry-Smith, MD Department of Emergency Medicine, McGovern School of Medicine, University of Texas Health Sciences Center at Houston, Houston, TX, USA

Ava E. Pierce, MD Department of Emergency Medicine, University of Texas Southwestern Medical Center, Dallas, TX, USA

Valerie A. Pierre, MD Department of Emergency Medicine, University of Maryland School of Medicine, Baltimore, MD, USA

Kiara Rogers, MD Department of Emergency Medicine, McGovern School of Medicine, University of Texas Health Sciences Center at Houston, Houston, TX, USA

Sangeeta S. Sakaria, MD, MPH, MST Department of Emergency Medicine, Cambridge Health Alliance, Cambridge, MA, USA

Pierre-Carole Tchouapi, MD Department of Emergency Medicine, State University of New York Downstate Health Sciences University, Brooklyn, NY, USA

Abbreviations

$G_xP_xA_x$	Gravida (number of pregnancies), Para (number of births of viable offspring), Abortus (number of abortions)
m	Meter
cm	Centimeter
mm	Millimeter
L	Liter
dL	Deciliter
mL	Milliliter
kg	Kilogram
g	Gram
C	Celsius
F	Fahrenheit
IU	International Units
miu	Milli-International–Units
h	Hour
min	Minute
GI	Gastrointestinal
IV	Intravenous
mmHg	Millimeters of mercury
U	Unit
mcg	Microgram
RBC	Red blood cell
WBC	White blood cell

Hyperemesis Gravidarum

Not Just Morning Sickness

Cassandra Bradby

Case

A 25-year-old woman, G1P0 at 5 weeks' gestational age, presents to the emergency department (ED) with a complaint of persistent nausea and vomiting. Earlier this week, she had a positive home pregnancy test and then visited her gynecologist requesting an evaluation for her first pregnancy with associated nausea and vomiting. She was given a prescription for ondansetron and discharged with instructions for care in the first trimester. The symptoms persisted, which led her to visit a local urgent care center. There, she was given a prescription for doxylamine/pyridoxine to alleviate symptoms. Today, she vomited over ten times and has been unable to tolerate fluids or solid food. The emesis has been non-bloody and non-bilious each time. Nothing, including the prescribed medications, has helped the symptoms. She notes that she has been more tired than usual this week and feels dehydrated. She denies fevers, chills, abdominal pain, chest pain, dizziness, or headache.

- Past medical history: None
- Past surgical history: None
- Medications: Prenatal vitamins, doxylamine/pyridoxine, ondansetron
- Allergies: No known drug allergies
- Family history: No pertinent family history
- Social history: No smoking, drinking of alcohol, or illicit drug use.

C. Bradby (✉)
Department of Emergency Medicine, East Carolina University Brody School of Medicine, Greenville, NC, USA
e-mail: bradbyc14@ecu.edu

© The Author(s), under exclusive license to Springer Nature Switzerland AG 2024
A. A. Kosoko (ed.), *Emergency Medicine Case-Based Guide*,
https://doi.org/10.1007/978-3-031-70118-4_1

Physical Exam

- Vital Signs

    - Heart rate: 110 beats/minute
    - Blood pressure: 105/82 mmHg
    - Respiratory rate: 16 breaths/minute
    - Temperature: 98.4 °F
    - Oxygen saturation: 100% on room air

- General appearance: Appears tired, lying back in the bed, in no acute distress. Emesis bag noted at the bedside, containing clear fluid
- HEENT

    - Head: Atraumatic, normocephalic
    - Eyes: Pupils equal, round, and reactive to light; normal extraocular movements; subconjunctival hemorrhage noted in the left eye
    - Throat: Dry mucous membranes
    - Neck: Trachea midline, no jugular venous distention present

- Heart: Tachycardia, regular rhythm, distal pulses equal bilaterally
- Lungs: Clear to auscultation bilaterally, speaks full sentences
- Abdominal/GI: Soft, nontender, not distended
- Genitourinary: Deferred
- Rectal: Deferred
- Extremities: No pedal edema, no tenderness
- Back: No costovertebral tenderness, no midline tenderness
- Neuro: Alert and oriented to person, place, and time; no focal neurological deficits
- Skin: Capillary refill is 3–4 seconds, no rashes
- Lymph: Normal
- Psych: No suicidal or homicidal ideation; normal thought processes; normal judgment

Pertinent Diagnostic Tests (Figs. 1.1 and 1.2, Tables 1.1, 1.2, 1.3, 1.4, 1.5, 1.6 and 1.7)

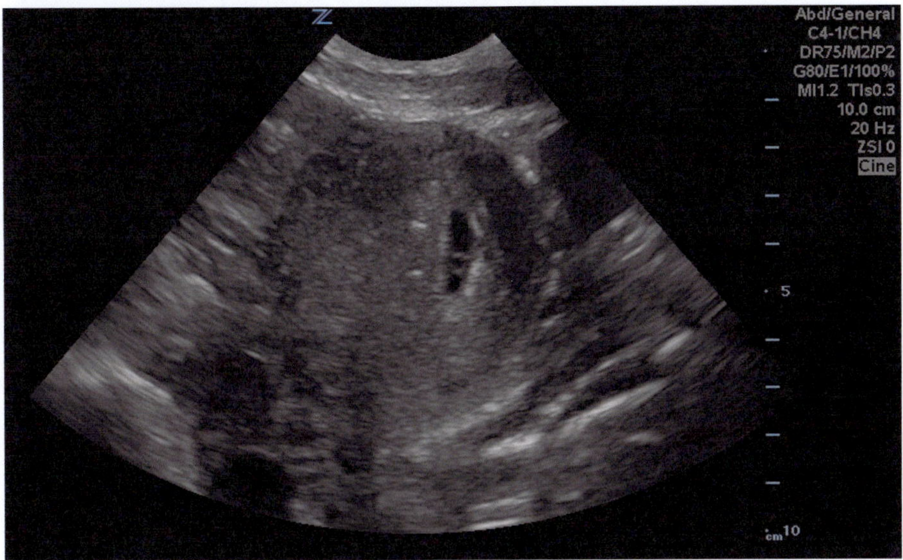

Fig. 1.1 Point of care pelvic ultrasound (POCUS): Early intrauterine pregnancy (Image provided by Kimberly Rathbun, MD and used with permission)

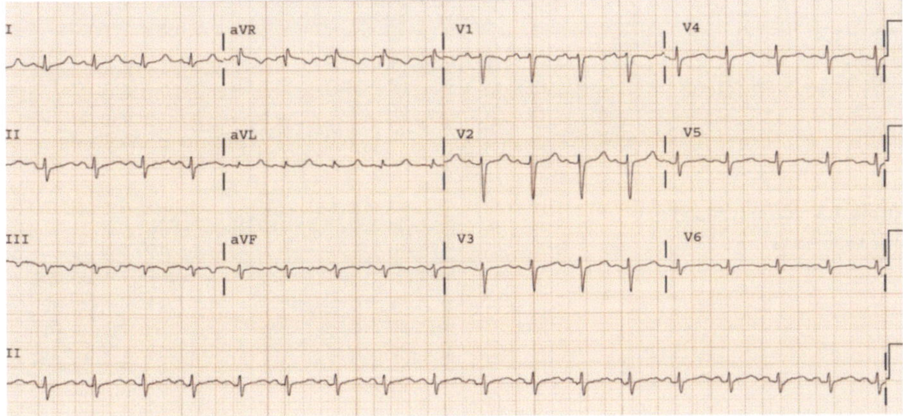

Fig. 1.2 Electrocardiogram (ECG): Sinus tachycardia, heart rate 101 beats/minute. (Author's own image)

Table 1.1 Complete blood count

Complete blood count	
White blood cells	15.9 x 10⁹/L
Hemoglobin	13.2 g/dL
Hematocrit	39.6%
Platelets	301 x 10⁹/L

Table 1.2 Comprehensive metabolic panel

Comprehensive metabolic panel	
Sodium	125 mEq/L
Potassium	2.7 mEq/L
Chloride	92 mEq/L
Bicarbonate	28 mEq/L
Glucose	90 mg/dL
Blood urea nitrogen (BUN)	70 mg/dL
Creatinine	2.01 mg/dL
Calcium	8.9 mg/dL
Total bilirubin	1.3 mg/dL
Alkaline phosphatase	121 units/L
Aspartate aminotransferase (AST)	30 units/L
Alanine aminotransferase (ALT)	31 units/L
Albumin	3.7 g/dL
Total protein	6.8 g/dL

Table 1.3 Serum magnesium and phosphorus

Additional electrolytes	
Magnesium	1.2 mg/dL
Phosphorus	1.8 mg/dL

Table 1.4 Thyroid function tests

Thyroid function tests		
TSH	<0.1 mIU/L	
Free T4	3.1 ng/dL	Reference range: 0.8–1.8 ng/dL

Table 1.5 Venous blood gas and lactic acid

Venous blood gas and lactic acid	
pH	7.53
pCO2	58 mmHg
pO2	105 mmHg
HCO3	27 mEq/L
Lactic acid	2.5 mEq/L

Table 1.6 β-human chorionic gonadotropin (β-hCG)

β-hCG	7451 mIU/mL

Table 1.7 Urinalysis

Urinalysis	
Color	Dark yellow
Appearance	Clear
Specific gravity	1.030
pH	7.55
Glucose	Negative
Bilirubin	Negative
Ketones	4+
Protein	Trace
Leukocyte esterase	Negative
Nitrites	Negative
White blood cells (WBC)	None
Red blood cells (RBC)	None
Squamous epithelial cells	None

Learning Points

Background

Nausea and vomiting in pregnancy are very common symptoms. However, when the symptoms progress to intractable nausea and vomiting with intravascular volume depletion, weight loss, electrolyte derangements, and ketone production, a diagnosis of hyperemesis gravidarum can be made [1]. When considering the spectrum of nausea and vomiting in pregnancy, hyperemesis gravidarum is on the most extreme end of the spectrum with the most severe symptoms. It occurs in approximately 0.3–2% of pregnancies worldwide, and the symptoms can be very difficult to control [2]. The average onset of symptoms is between 5 and 6 weeks of pregnancy.

There are multiple hypotheses regarding contributing factors in the development of hyperemesis. These include responses to elevated hormones (human chorionic gonadotropin (hCG), progesterone, estrogen, and thyroid hormone); presence of *Helicobacter pylori*; decreased lower esophageal sphincter tone and gastroesophageal reflux; and genetic factors. Women who are more prone to experiencing nausea and vomiting for any reason outside of pregnancy are at higher risk for hyperemesis gravidarum. No single cause of hyperemesis has been found [3].

Populations with higher prevalence of hyperemesis gravidarum include those with gestational trophoblastic disease, pregnancies with multiple gestations, and those with family history of hyperemesis gravidarum.

Identification of hyperemesis gravidarum is important due to its risk for significant morbidity and mortality for both mother and fetus. Prolonged hyperemesis gravidarum can lead to severe electrolyte derangements, arrhythmias, and even Wernicke's encephalopathy.

Differential Diagnosis gestational trophoblastic disease, multiple gestation pregnancy, peptic ulcer disease, gastritis, acute fatty liver of pregnancy, thyrotoxicosis, HELLP (hemolysis, elevated liver function tests, low platelets) syndrome, pancreatitis, pyelonephritis.

History and Physical Exam

Patients will present with a chief complaint of intractable nausea and vomiting in the first trimester of pregnancy. They may also have fatigue or weight loss. In severe cases, patients may have jaundice secondary to liver dysfunction.

History-taking should identify the estimated gestational age, how many fetuses are present (if known), and prior pregnancies including any associated complications. The vomiting episodes should be described as best as the patient is able including timing, frequency, color, severity, and any interventions tried. Most cases of hyperemesis gravidarum are present in the first trimester, around weeks 5 or 6 of gestation. Most cases subside by 20 weeks of gestation, though a minority of patients will continue to have nausea and vomiting into the third trimester. If abdominal pain is a dominant symptom described by the patient, hyperemesis gravidarum is less likely the primary diagnosis, and other diagnoses should be pursued with more scrutiny.

The physical exam should include a full set of vital signs to evaluate for hypovolemic shock typically presenting with tachycardia and hypotension. The weight of the patient should be obtained to evaluate trends of improvement or worsening condition. A weight loss of more than 5% of pre-pregnancy weight is highly suggestive of hyperemesis gravidarum.

Other markers of hydration status should be evaluated, including mucus membranes, capillary refill, and skin turgor. Abdominal or pelvic tenderness is not typically observed when diagnosing hyperemesis gravidarum.

The modified Pregnancy-Unique Quantification of Emesis and Nausea (PUQE) score is a validated objective scoring system used to assess the severity of nausea and vomiting. The score correlates well with the risk of hospitalization in a pregnant patient. It relies on three questions (Table 1.8). A score greater than or equal to 13 indicates hyperemesis gravidarum [4].

Table 1.8 The modified Pregnancy-Unique Quantification of Emesis and Nausea (PUQE) score

Questions	1	2	3	4	5
In the last 24 hours, for how long have you felt nauseated or sick to your stomach?	Not at all	<1 hour	1 to 3 hours	3 to 6 hours	>6 hours
In the last 24 hours, how many times have you vomited or thrown-up?	None	1 to 2	3 to 4	5 to 6	≥7
In the last 24 hours, how many times have you had retching or dry heaving without throwing up?	Not at all	1 to 2	3 to 4	5 to 6	≥7

Laboratory Studies

Hyperemesis gravidarum is a clinical diagnosis. However, the presence of ketones in the blood or urine in a patient with vomiting is highly suggestive of hyperemesis gravidarum. Other laboratory studies which may be obtained would be to evaluate for complications of high volume, high frequency emesis, and anorexia or to evaluate for other items on the differential diagnosis.

Investigation of this condition should include a comprehensive metabolic panel with magnesium and phosphorus, to assess for electrolyte derangements, renal injury, and liver dysfunction. Hyponatremia and hypokalemia are common signs of voluminous vomiting. A severely elevated BUN:creatinine ratio can indicate that acute renal injury has occurred due to dehydration. A complete blood count showing an elevated hemoglobin or hematocrit level can suggest decreased intravascular volume (hemoconcentration). Urinalysis can suggest dehydration by an elevated specific gravity, a sign of volume depletion. Elevated ketones in the urine or in the serum often reflect poor nutritional intake and resultant breakdown of the body's fat stores for energy. Additional labs such as thyroid function tests, liver enzymes, and lipase should be obtained to assess for alternative diagnoses. A β-hCG level is useful for understanding whether there is concern for gestational trophoblastic disease or for multiple fetuses.

Acid–base status in patients with hyperemesis can vary. Most commonly these patients have metabolic alkalosis from the loss of stomach acid during vomiting. In addition, hypochloremia, hypokalemia, and hypovolemia exacerbate the reabsorption of bicarbonate ions as the body attempts to maintain electrochemical neutrality by increasing aldosterone levels [5]. However, should vomiting be severe enough, it can lead to metabolic acidosis due to starvation ketosis. Lactic acidosis in pregnancy is usually pathologic, most concerning for reflecting various causes of shock. When the mother is in shock, perfusion to the fetus can be one of the first compromised areas of perfusion in the body. Elevated lactic acid levels in pregnancy should be treated according to the suspected cause [6].

It is also notable that up to two-thirds of patients with hyperemesis gravidarum also have transient hyperthyroidism, demonstrating depressed TSH levels and elevated free T4 levels. It is believed that the elevation of serum hCG contributes to this phenomenon because the hCG molecule is structurally similar to the TSH molecule and may activate T4 production. Free T4 levels usually normalize by 15 weeks of gestation, after which the patients typically do not have clinical signs of hyperthyroidism [7]. If the patient presents with signs of clinical hyperthyroidism, (e.g., goiter and heart rate greater than 120 beats/minute, protruding eyes, etc.), Graves' disease and other thyroid dysfunction should be considered.

Imaging Findings

There is no formal imaging required for the diagnosis of hyperemesis gravidarum. However, if no ultrasound has been obtained during the pregnancy to date, an obstetric ultrasound should be obtained to assess for an intrauterine pregnancy, multiple gestations, or gestational trophoblastic disease. An ultrasound will also reassure against an ectopic pregnancy and ensure that the fetus has remained viable despite the stress from vomiting afflicting the mother.

An ECG should be obtained to evaluate whether severe electrolyte derangements are adversely affecting the myocardium.

Management

Emergency department management should be focused on volume repletion and management of symptoms. Intravenous (IV) fluids that include dextrose help with the treatment of dehydration and clearing ketonuria/ketonemia, ceasing body fat breakdown due to starvation. It may be beneficial to administer parenteral thiamine before glucose to prevent the development of Wernicke's encephalopathy. It is also recommended to correct hypokalemia prior to administering glucose. Theoretically, hypokalemia can be worsened by the insulin release stimulated by the increased serum dextrose levels because insulin drives potassium into cells. If IV access is difficult to obtain, nasogastric fluid (electrolyte containing or oral rehydration solution) and nutrition resuscitation can be considered. Any electrolyte derangements should be corrected. When intravenous fluids are needed, intravenous antiemetics are usually needed to prevent further nausea and vomiting (Table 1.9). Medications such as ondansetron, metoclopramide, promethazine, and chlorpromazine can be given to help with nausea.

If a patient is being discharged home, nausea and vomiting can be managed by using folic acid supplementation instead of typical prenatal vitamins and considering ginger supplementation in food, drink, or by tablets. Prescriptions for pyridoxine (vitamin B6) and doxylamine are the United States Food and Drug Administration (FDA) pregnancy Category A medications. The only drug currently approved by the FDA for nausea and vomiting in pregnancy is doxylamine-pyridoxine. If taken at bedtime, the drug achieves optimum serum levels in the morning, when nausea and vomiting tend to be worst for many pregnant patients.

Antihistamine agents and anti-dopaminergic agents act as second-line medications for refractory cases.

Table 1.9 Antiemetic agents and dosing recommendations

Drug	Dosage	Frequency	FDA pregnancy rating
Pyridoxine (vitamin B6)	10–25 mg	Every 6–8 h	A
Doxylamine	12.5 mg	Every 6–8 h	A
Dimenhydrinate	25–50 mg	Every 4–6 h	B
Diphenhydramine	25–50 mg	Every 4–6 h	B
Ondansetron	4–8 mg	Every 4 h	B
Metoclopramide	5–10 mg	Every 8 h	B
Prochlorperazine	5–10 mg	Every 6–8 h oral or IV	C
	25 mg	Every 12 h rectal	
Promethazine	12.5–25 mg	Every 4–6 h oral or rectal	C

FDA United States food and drug administration

Methylprednisolone may be used as an adjunct therapy for refractory cases (16 mg parenterally or orally every 8 hours for 3 days).

Severe cases of hyperemesis gravidarum should be admitted for rehydration, nutrition supplementation, and electrolyte management. If a patient is not able to tolerate oral intake, a hospital admission is indicated.

Consultation Considerations

An obstetrician/gynecologist will be the optimal consultant for inpatient management of hyperemesis gravidarum. Even if the patient is to be discharged, close obstetric/gynecologic follow-up should be ensured for optimal outcomes of the mother and baby.

For severe cases of hyperemesis gravidarum, a mental health consultation (psychiatry, psychology) may be indicated to help with behavior modification or for depressive symptoms that can result from the condition.

Emergency Department Course and Outcome

The patient was moderately dehydrated and had another episode of emesis during her initial evaluation. Intravenous access was obtained peripherally, and she received metoclopramide and one liter of normal saline. She unfortunately had another episode of retching when the nurses tried to encourage oral intake after her fluids had completely been administered. She continued to have an elevated heart rate of 108 beats/minute. Another liter of IV normal saline was administered. Once the tachycardia resolved, a normal saline solution of dextrose 5% and potassium chloride (D5NS + 40 mEq KCl) was infused at 1.5 times maintenance rate to assist in clearing her ketonemia/ketonuria.

While the patient was in the ED, she had only urinated once for the urinalysis and had failed to tolerate oral intake. The obstetrics/gynecology team was consulted for continued inpatient management.

During her 3-day hospital stay, the patient tried various multimodal combinations to combat her nausea, while receiving IV fluids. She started urinating regularly, her heart rate normalized, she was no longer experiencing ketonemia, and she was feeling much better. Ultimately, she started taking small amounts of bland foods, utilizing ginger candies and teas throughout the day, along with scheduled pyridoxine. She was prescribed ondansetron oral disintegrating tablets for use with exacerbation of her condition and rectal promethazine for when her symptoms were refractory. The patient understood the benefits and the potential risks of the use of the agents she was prescribed. She was discharged home in good condition and with an appointment for a reassessment of her weight and overall progress in 5 days with her obstetrician.

Key Points

- The modified Pregnancy-Unique Quantification of Emesis and Nausea (PUQE) score is a validated objective scoring system to help identify routine nausea and vomiting of pregnancy from hyperemesis gravidarum.
- Fluid resuscitation, antiemetics, and electrolyte repletion are the mainstays of management of hyperemesis gravidarum.
- Dextrose-containing IV fluids are often needed to help interrupt ketosis present with hyperemesis gravidarum.
- Consider other diagnoses if abdominal pain or additional symptoms beyond nausea and vomiting is present.

References

1. Committee on Practice Bulletins-Obstetrics. ACOG Practice Bulletin No. 189: nausea and vomiting of pregnancy. Obstet Gynecol. 2018;131(1):e15–30. https://doi.org/10.1097/AOG.0000000000002456.
2. Philip B. Hyperemesis gravidarum: literature review. WMJ. 2003;102(3):46–51.
3. Austin K, Wilson K, Saha S. Hyperemesis Gravidarum. Nutr Clin Pract. 2019;34(2):226–41. https://doi.org/10.1002/ncp.10205.
4. Lacasse A, Rey E, Ferreira E, Morin C, Bérard A. Validity of a modified pregnancy-unique quantification of emesis and nausea (PUQE) scoring index to assess severity of nausea and vomiting of pregnancy. Am J Obstet Gynecol. 2008;198(1):e1–7. https://doi.org/10.1016/j.ajog.2007.05.051.
5. Frise C, Noori M, Williamson C. Severe metabolic alkalosis in pregnancy. Obstet Med. 2013;6(3):138–40. https://doi.org/10.1258/om.2012.120030.
6. Ahmed A. Fetomaternal acid-base balance and electrolytes during pregnancy. Indian J Crit Care Med. 2021;25(Suppl 3):S193–9. https://doi.org/10.5005/jp-journals-10071-24030.
7. Tan JY, Loh KC, Yeo GS, Chee YC. Transient hyperthyroidism of hyperemesis gravidarum. BJOG. 2002;109(6):683–8. https://doi.org/10.1111/j.1471-0528.2002.01223.x.

Ectopic Pregnancy

Location. Location. Location.

Suchismita Datta

Case

A 32-year-old woman presents with a complaint of abdominal pain and lighthead-edness. The patient explains that she began feeling pain in her right lower abdomen which began a few hours ago but has been worsening. She has never experienced anything like this before. She has nausea associated with the pain, but there is no vomiting or diarrhea. She denies any chest pain but felt like it was harder to breathe when walking earlier. There is no vaginal bleeding, discharge, or urinary symptoms. Over the last 30 minutes, she has felt more lightheaded and weaker. Upon standing from her seated position to get into her examination bed, she felt dizzy.

- Past medical history: G2P2 (normal spontaneous vaginal deliveries), pelvic inflammatory disease as a teenager
- Past surgical history: None
- Medications: Contraceptive injection, vitamin supplements
- Allergies: No known drug allergies
- Family history: Mother has diabetes, father has hypertension
- Social history: Non-smoker, drinks alcohol occasionally

Supplementary Information The online version contains supplementary material available at https://doi.org/10.1007/978-3-031-70118-4_2.

S. Datta (✉)
Department of Emergency Medicine, New York University Grossman Long Island School of Medicine, Mineola, NY, USA
e-mail: suchismita.datta@nyulangone.org

Physical Exam

- Vital signs
  - Heart rate: 122 beats/minute
  - Blood pressure: 83/53
  - Respiratory rate: 22 breaths/minute
  - Temperature: 97.2 °F
  - Oxygen saturation: 97% on room air
- General appearance: Appears stated age, pale, lying in bed, in obvious distress secondary to pain
- HEENT
  - Head: Atraumatic, normocephalic
  - Eyes: Pupils equal, round, and reactive to light (4–2 mm); external ocular movements are normal; normal conjunctiva; no papilledema
  - Ears: Normal
  - Nose: Normal
  - Throat: No erythema or edema of the oropharynx
  - Neck: Trachea midline, no stridor
- Heart: Tachycardia, regular rhythm, equal pulses
- Lungs: No respiratory distress, speaks full sentences without difficulty, clear to auscultation
- Abdominal/GI: Soft, diffusely tender with rebound tenderness and guarding, bowel sounds present
- Genitourinary: Normal external, no vaginal bleeding, internal exam deferred
- Rectal: Normal
- Extremities: No edema, no tenderness, no deformity, full range of motion intact bilateral upper and lower extremities
- Back: Normal
- Neuro: Alert, oriented, normal reflexes, normal strength, grossly normal coordination
- Skin: Cool, mildly diaphoretic
- Lymph: Normal
- Psych: Slightly anxious, otherwise normal

Pertinent Diagnostic Tests (Figs. 2.1, 2.2 a,b,c, and 2.3, Tables 2.1, 2.2, 2.3, 2.4, 2.5, 2.6 and 2.7)

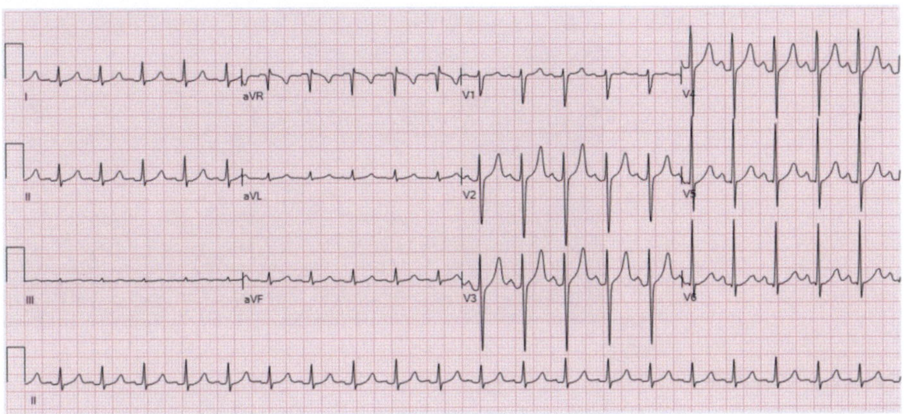

Fig. 2.1 Electrocardiogram (ECG): Sinus tachycardia. Nonspecific T-wave abnormalities. (Author's own image)

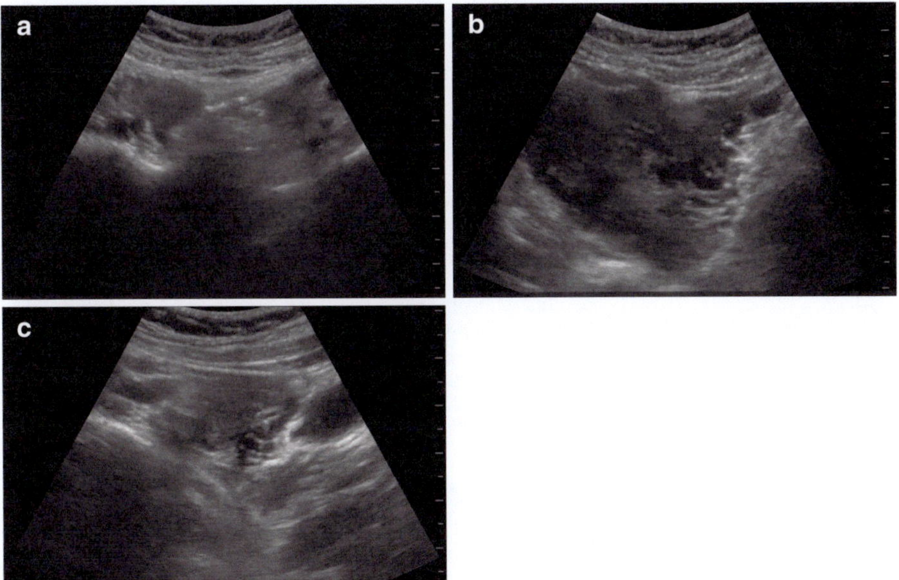

Fig. 2.2 Point-of-Care Pelvic Ultrasound, (**a**) Long uterus view, (**b**) Short uterus view, (**c**) Adnexa: No intrauterine pregnancy identified in uterus, abnormal adnexa. (Images courtesy of C. Bakunas, MD and R. Bower)

Fig. 2.3 Focused Abdominal Sonography in Trauma Exam: Fluid in right upper quadrant Morrison's pouch. (Images courtesy of C. Bakunas and R. Bower)

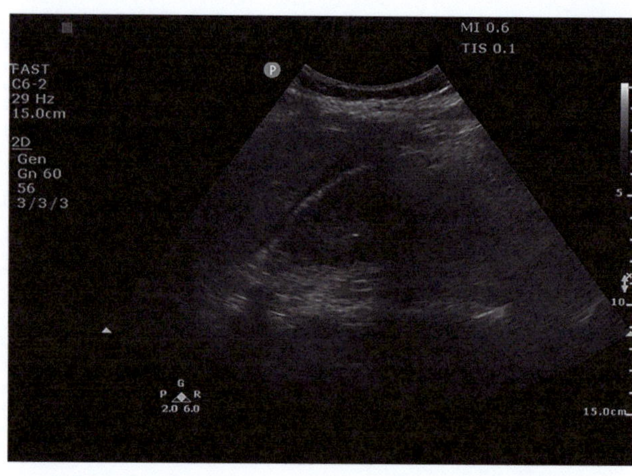

Table 2.1 Complete blood count

Complete blood count	
White blood cells	18 x 10⁹/L
Hemoglobin	9 g/dL
Hematocrit	22%
Platelets	240 x 10⁹/L

Table 2.2 Comprehensive metabolic panel

Comprehensive metabolic panel	
Sodium	136 mEq/L
Potassium	4.1 mEq/L
Chloride	109 mEq/L
Bicarbonate	24 mEq/L
Glucose	90 mg/dL
Blood urea nitrogen (BUN)	48 mg/dL
Creatinine	0.9 mg/dL
Calcium	9.0 mg/dL
Total bilirubin	0.5 mg/dL
Alkaline phosphatase	45 units/L
Aspartate aminotransferase (AST)	35 units/L
Alanine aminotransferase (ALT)	40 units/L
Albumin	3.7 g/dL
Total protein	6.8 g/dL

Table 2.3 Venous blood gas and lactic acid

Venous blood gas and lactic acid	
pH	7.37
pCO2	47.4 mmHg
pO2	35.1 mmHg
HCO3	25.2 mEq/L
Lactic acid	1.8 mEq/L

Table 2.4 Coagulopathy panel

Coagulopathy panel	
International normalized ratio (INR)	1.0
Prothrombin time (PT)	11.7 seconds
Activated partial thromboplastin time (aPTT)	29.6 seconds

Table 2.5 Blood type

Blood type	
ABO type	O
Rh(D) antigen	+

Table 2.6 Troponin I

Troponin I	< 0.04 ng/mL

Table 2.7 Urinalysis

Urinalysis (UA)	
Color	Yellow
Appearance	Clear
Specific gravity	1.010
pH	7.0
Glucose	Negative
Bilirubin	Negative
Ketones	0
Protein	1+
Leukocyte esterase	1+
Nitrites	Negative
White blood cells (WBCs)	1 WBC/High-Power Field (HPF)
Red blood cells (RBCs)	0 RBCs/HPF
Squamous epithelial cells	0–5 cells/HPF

Learning Points

Background

An ectopic pregnancy occurs when a fertilized egg implants outside of the uterus or in weakened areas of the uterus where there is scarred tissue. The fallopian tube is the most common location for ectopic pregnancy, accounting for roughly 90% of cases [1]. Other locations for ectopic pregnancy include the abdomen (1%), cervix (1%), ovary (1–3%), and cesarean scar (1–3%) [1]. The greatest risk factors for ectopic pregnancy are a history of ectopic pregnancy and a previous injury to the fallopian tubes (e.g., surgical procedures, pelvic inflammatory disease) [2, 3]. Women with history of ectopic pregnancy have a ten-fold increased chance of developing another ectopic pregnancy. Other risk factors include advanced maternal age, smoking, and assisted reproductive technology use.

An intrauterine pregnancy with a concurrent pregnancy outside of the uterus is called a heterotopic pregnancy. Heterotopic pregnancies are rare in the general population, but the risk of such pregnancies increase to as high as 1% among women who have undergone in vitro fertilization [2].

An ectopic pregnancy is not a viable pregnancy. The embryo will not be able to grow normally at the site of implantation, and a fetus cannot be sustained. Furthermore, as it grows, it can cause local structural damage which can lead to life-threatening maternal hemorrhage or infection. Ruptured ectopic pregnancies account for 2.7% of all pregnancy-related mortality and morbidity [4].

Differential Diagnosis Early normal intrauterine pregnancy, heterotopic pregnancy, ovarian torsion, appendicitis, spontaneous abortion.

History and Physical Exam

Ectopic pregnancies can have a wide range of presentations, including syncope, lower back pain, nausea and vomiting, vaginal bleeding, or even fatigue. However, most patients will have chief complaints of pelvic pain or abdominal pain. A positive home pregnancy test or other confirmatory test of a pregnant state is useful to guide the workup. The patient's last known menstrual period should be documented as well as whether she is using any form of birth control. If the patient is having pain, the onset and quality of pain will help in locating any potential ectopic pregnancy. If the patient is having vaginal bleeding, she should try to quantify her loss. Because a great risk factor for ectopic pregnancy is a previous ectopic pregnancy, it may even be useful to ask the patient outright if she has ever had an ectopic pregnancy before. Similarly, a patient should explicitly be asked if she has undergone any assistive reproductive treatments, some of which could place her at higher risk for ectopic or heterotopic pregnancy.

A full set of vital signs should be recorded. Tachycardia or hypotension could represent occult hemorrhage shock, which might occur in cases of ruptured ectopic pregnancy. A proper abdominal exam with the patient lying prone should be performed. Any tenderness elicited by palpation should be noted. Any peritoneal signs could be suggestive of blood in the peritoneum due to a ruptured ectopic pregnancy. A pelvic exam is useful to evaluate for other items on a differential diagnosis, including cervicitis or pelvic inflammatory disease or even a spontaneous abortion. However, though a larger uterus can suggest a pregnancy, it cannot affirm a normal intrauterine pregnancy. A bimanual exam can localize tenderness in the adnexa or at the uterus.

There should be a high index of suspicion for a ruptured ectopic pregnancy when a patient is hemodynamically unstable and in a known early pregnant state.

Laboratory Studies

Regardless of reported sexual activity, last known menstrual period, use of contraception, or report of pregnant state, every female who has the capability of getting pregnant should be tested for pregnancy. A urine pregnancy test is an adequate screen. A serum β-human chorionic gonadotropin (β-hCG) level can be obtained as a quantitative or qualitative test. A quantitative β-hCG level expectantly rises with gestational age in a normal pregnancy. The "discriminatory zone" is the term used to describe the β-hCG level at which an intrauterine pregnancy is expected to be visualized consistently by ultrasonography. Historically, abdominal ultrasound should identify an intrauterine pregnancy by gestational sac when the β-hCG level is greater than 6500 mIU/mL. A transvaginal (intracavitary) ultrasound should be used when the β-hCG level is higher than 1500 mIU/mL but the pregnancy cannot be identified using an abdominal ultrasound. The likelihood of successfully identifying a pregnancy when the β-hCG level is less than 1500 mIU/mL is low. However, more recently, the value of the discriminatory zone has been challenged [2, 5]. An inability to identify a gestational sac with a β-hCG level greater than 6500 mIU/mL is concerning for an ectopic pregnancy. However, it is best to approach the patient's serum β-hCG level as a trend rather than a single point of information [2]. If a definitive intrauterine pregnancy is not identified, the serum β-hCG should be measured again in two days and should be about double the previous value at reassessment. Serum β-hCG levels typically increase in a curvilinear fashion and plateau at 100,000 mIU/mL. Decreasing β-hCG levels can suggest that the pregnancy is failing; however, this alone is not considered diagnostic and should be monitored until nonpregnant levels are reached [2].

Other important laboratory tests to consider are to evaluate for significant hemorrhage (i.e., hemoglobin and hematocrit) and signs of coagulopathy (i.e., platelet count, coagulation studies). A blood type and screen would prepare for a blood transfusion and determine if the patient needs to receive $Rh_o(D)$ immune globulin to protect any future pregnancies.

Imaging Findings

Ultrasonography is the mainstay of diagnosis of ectopic pregnancy. The pelvic ultrasound is best used with a serum β-hCG level to best interpret findings. Transvaginal ultrasound provides the highest resolution images, but as a pregnancy has progressed, an abdominal ultrasound may provide sufficient imaging of products of conception. The major question that should be asked when performing a first trimester ultrasound is "Is there an intrauterine pregnancy (yolk sac, fetal pole, fetal heartbeat)?" A gestational sac alone cannot qualify as an intrauterine pregnancy, as 10–20% of ectopic pregnancies also have a gestational sac (pseudogestational sac) [6]. The preferred standard for diagnosing an intrauterine pregnancy is by visualizing cardiac activity. However, definitive ultrasonography evidence of intrauterine pregnancy can be acquired at as early as 5 weeks of gestation (Fig. 2.4).

If a patient's laboratory tests suggest pregnancy but there is any mass identified at the adnexa with a hypoechoic area separate from the ovary, an ectopic pregnancy should be suspected [2, 7].

Identifying an intrauterine pregnancy will typically rule out an ectopic pregnancy, unless the patient has a rare case of heterotopic pregnancy. Half of heterotopic cases are only diagnosed upon medical complications identified with progression of the condition.

However, if β-hCG level suggests a pregnancy and an intrauterine pregnancy cannot be identified on ultrasound, one of three diagnostic outcomes is possible:

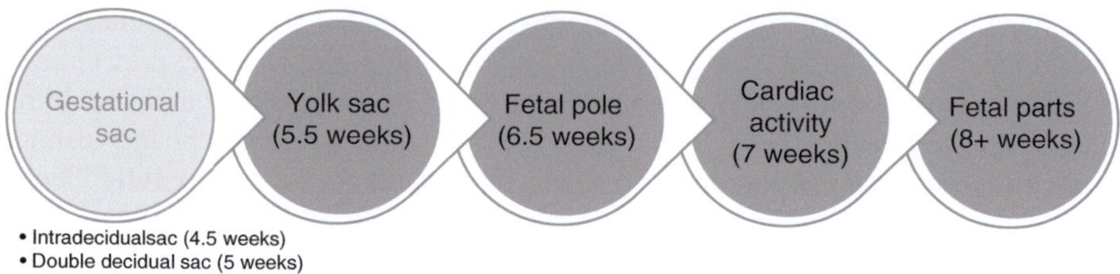

Fig. 2.4 Expected progression of ultrasound findings for an intrauterine pregnancy

there was a missed or complete spontaneous abortion, the pregnancy is too early to determine exactly what is occurring and will need to be reassessed, or the pregnancy is an ectopic pregnancy. The history and physical exam will help determine which of these outcomes is most likely for the patient.

Management

The unstable patient should immediately be resuscitated with primary focus on the airway, breathing, and circulation. A clinically unstable patient is most likely the result of a ruptured ectopic pregnancy and subsequent hemorrhagic shock. However, most patients will be generally stable, presenting with pain or mild vaginal bleeding.

Management decisions are based on the patient's clinical status, the β-hCG level, and the ultrasound findings, including size of the embryo. Decisions should be made with the patient based on her preference but also based on her outpatient resources.

Medical management is the preferred approach to addressing an intact ectopic pregnancy in a hemodynamically stable patient. Methotrexate, a folic acid antagonist, interferes with cell proliferation. It is the safest and most studied agent, and its use is based on good and consistent scientific evidence from the American College of Obstetricians and Gynecologists [2]. Methotrexate is an option when the ectopic pregnancy is small (<3.5 cm diameter) and works best with β-hCG levels less than 1500 mIU/mL [8]. β-hCG levels greater than 5000 mIU/mL are least likely to respond to methotrexate as a therapy. The dose of methotrexate given for an ectopic pregnancy is low compared to the dose used for other indications (e.g., chemotherapy), which limits the side effects of nausea, vomiting, or diarrhea. Single dose methotrexate is effective in 71% of cases, and efficacy of methotrexate increases up to 94% with the addition of a second dose [9, 10]. One approach is to administer one dose of intramuscular methotrexate 50 mg/m^2, then recheck the β-hCG level 4 to 7 days later to determine whether another dose of methotrexate should be administered. Methotrexate should not be given if there is a fetal heartbeat, the embryo is >3.5 cm in diameter, the β-hCG level is more than 5000 mIU/mL or if there is suspected ruptured ectopic pregnancy. It should not be given to women who have significant liver disease or renal disease.

A meta-analysis of four randomized clinical trials suggested that when comparing methotrexate and expectant management for treatment success (defined as declining beta hCG levels) in hemodynamically stable patients with low or declining beta hCG levels, the difference was statistically insignificant. The same study also found that the difference in need for surgical intervention between the two treatment modalities was also statistically insignificant [11]. The decision to pursue expectant management from the ED would require a reliable patient and dependable circumstances.

A comparative review of major guidelines showed that there is consensus agreement across multiple obstetric/gynecologic societies that laparoscopy is the optimal surgical technique for patients who are hemodynamically stable [12]. Salpingectomy is presently more common than salpingostomy in the effort to optimally preserve future fertility. Laparotomy should be restricted to patients who have ruptured ectopic pregnancies, have excessive bleeding, are hemodynamically unstable, or have advanced abdominal pregnancy with placenta attached to major vessels [12]. Unfortunately, surgical interventions can increase risk of future ectopic pregnancies.

Consultation Considerations

An emergency gynecologist consultation is necessary for any patient for whom a ruptured ectopic pregnancy is suspected because these patients will need surgical intervention.

Most ectopic pregnancy cases will be managed medically with methotrexate. Most of these cases will be managed in an outpatient setting. A gynecologist can assist in navigating decisions about methotrexate administration and dosing. Most importantly, the patient will need close outpatient care with a gynecologist to determine the efficacy of any medical management.

Emergency Department Course and Outcome

The emergency team administered a two-liter bolus of isotonic intravenous fluids and gave fentanyl to manage the patient's pain. The emergency physician performed a point-of-care pelvic and abdomen ultrasound and identified a small strip of fluid at Morrison's pouch. Though the uterus had a gestational sac, there was no yolk sac identified. A serum quantitative β-hCG level was 95,000 mIU/mL. An emergency consultation was made to the gynecology team with concern for a ruptured ectopic pregnancy.

While waiting for the consultant's evaluation, the patient complained of increased abdominal pain and her blood pressure read 78/49 mmHg with a heart rate of 122 beats/minute. Emergency blood products were released with concern for hemorrhagic shock, and the patient received one unit of type O-negative packed red blood cells given with a rapid transfuser.

Upon arrival of the consultants, a repeat point-of care ultrasound of the pelvis confirmed peritoneal blood. The decision was to take the patient emergently for surgical exploration.

Key Points

- The number one question to ask when performing a pelvic ultrasound is whether an intrauterine pregnancy exists. If there is any uncertainty to the answer, an ectopic pregnancy has not been ruled out.
- The discriminatory zone based on β-hCG levels may be useful to determine which ultrasound probe to use to identify an intrauterine pregnancy; however, the values are merely guidelines. If a yolk sac cannot be seen above a threshold value, evaluation must continue in an organized fashion to determine whether an intrauterine pregnancy or an ectopic pregnancy exists.
- Medical management with methotrexate for an early ectopic pregnancy is safe and effective. However, contraindications to methotrexate must first be considered.
- Heterotopic pregnancies are rare but are more likely to occur in patients undergoing reproductive assistance. The expertise of an obstetrician or gynecologist is often needed to help thoroughly evaluate for a heterotopic pregnancy.

References

1. Bouyer J, Coste J, Fernandez H, Pouly JL, Job-Spira N. Sites of ectopic pregnancy: a 10 year population-based study of 1800 cases. Hum Reprod. 2002;17(12):3224–30. https://doi.org/10.1093/humrep/17.12.3224.
2. American College of Obstetricians and Gynecologists' Committee on Practice Bulletins—Gynecology. ACOG practice bulletin no. 193: tubal ectopic pregnancy. Obstet Gynecol. 2018;131(3):e91–e103. https://doi.org/10.1097/AOG.0000000000002560. Erratum in: Obstet Gynecol. 2019 May;133(5):1059
3. Barnhart KT, Sammel MD, Gracia CR, Chittams J, Hummel AC, Shaunik A. Risk factors for ectopic pregnancy in women with symptomatic first-trimester pregnancies. Fertil Steril. 2006;86(1):36–43. https://doi.org/10.1016/j.fertnstert.2005.12.023.
4. Creanga AA, Syverson C, Seed K, Callaghan WM. Pregnancy-related mortality in the United States, 2011-2013. Obstet Gynecol. 2017;130(2):366–73. https://doi.org/10.1097/AOG.0000000000002114.
5. Fu J, Henne MB, Blumstein SL, Lathi RB. Ruptured ectopic pregnancy with minimally detectable Beta-HCG level. Fertil Steril. 2005;83(5):s25–6. https://doi.org/10.1016/j.fertnstert.2005.01.063.
6. Yeh HC, Goodman JD, Carr L, Rabinowitz JG. Intradecidual sign: a US criterion of early intrauterine pregnancy. Radiology. 1986;161(2):463–7. https://doi.org/10.1148/radiology.161.2.3532191.
7. Barnhart KT, Fay CA, Suescum M, Sammel MD, Appleby D, Shaunik A, Dean AJ. Clinical factors affecting the accuracy of ultrasonography in symptomatic first-trimester pregnancy. Obstet Gynecol. 2011;117(2 Pt 1):299–306. https://doi.org/10.1097/AOG.0b013e3182050ed0.

8. Corsan GH, Karacan M, Qasim S, Bohrer MK, Ransom MX, Kemmann E. Identification of hormonal parameters for successful systemic single-dose methotrexate therapy in ectopic pregnancy. Hum Reprod. 1995;10(10):2719–22. https://doi.org/10.1093/oxfordjournals.humrep.a135774.
9. Stovall TG, Ling FW. Single-dose methotrexate: an expanded clinical trial. Am J Obstet Gynecol. 1993;168(6 Pt 1):1759–62.; discussion 1762-5. https://doi.org/10.1016/0002-9378(93)90687-e.
10. Parker J, Bisits A, Proietto AM. A systematic review of single-dose intramuscular methotrexate for the treatment of ectopic pregnancy. Aust N Z J Obstet Gynaecol. 1998;38(2):145–50. https://doi.org/10.1111/j.1479-828x.1998.tb02988.x.
11. Naveed AK, Anjum MU, Hassan A, Mahmood SN. Methotrexate versus expectant management in ectopic pregnancy: a meta-analysis. Arch Gynecol Obstet. 2022;305(3):547–53. https://doi.org/10.1007/s00404-021-06236-y.
12. Tsakiridis I, Giouleka S, Mamopoulos A, Athanasiadis A, Dagklis T. Diagnosis and management of ectopic pregnancy: a comparative review of major National Guidelines. Obstet Gynecol Surv. 2020;75(10):611–23. https://doi.org/10.1097/OGX.0000000000000832.

Gestational Trophoblastic Disease

Beta Think Twice

3

Omoyeni O. Clement and Adeola A. Kosoko

Case

A 29-year-old G5P2022 woman at 2 weeks and 1 day gestational age, as measured by last menstrual period, presents to the emergency department (ED) with a chief complaint of pain in her abdomen and chest. The pain has been present for 8 days and is localized to the left upper abdomen and left lower chest region. Her pain is 9 out of 10 in severity, improved when sitting up compared to lying flat. Five days ago, she was having episodes of malodorous vaginal discharge for which she received an evaluation in a community clinic. She was diagnosed with a urinary tract infection (UTI) and was discharged on ciprofloxacin and dicycloverine.

Two days prior to her ED presentation, she again went to another outside hospital for continued pain with unchanged quality but with a new associated cough. Her documentation for that visit noted rales on the physical exam and a β-human chorionic gonadotropin (β-hCG) level of 119,538 mIU/mL. A chest radiograph showed interstitial infiltrates and peribronchial cuffing, concerning for atypical pneumonia. A computed tomography angiography (CTA) of the chest was obtained, demonstrating consolidative infiltrates peripherally in the lingula and bilateral lower lobes and trace bilateral pleural effusions. Although there was no lung mass or acute pulmonary embolus, there were some fatty infiltrations of the liver. The patient was diagnosed with multifocal pneumonia and discharged from the facility with a prescription for amoxicillin-clavulanate.

Supplementary Information The online version contains supplementary material available at https://doi.org/10.1007/978-3-031-70118-4_3.

O. O. Clement · A. A. Kosoko (✉)
Department of Emergency Medicine, McGovern School of Medicine, University of Texas Health Sciences Center at Houston, Houston, TX, USA
e-mail: Adeola.A.Kosoko@uth.tmc.edu

Today, she laments that she simply does not feel better, despite adhering to the instructions of the two antibiotic regimens and her analgesia.

- Past medical history: None
- Obstetric history: 2 prior spontaneous abortions, 2 term live births. Molar pregnancy three years prior treated by dilation and curettage (D&C).
- Past surgical history: D&C 3 years ago
- Medications: Ciprofloxacin, dicycloverine, amoxicillin-clavulanate
- Allergies: None
- Family history: None pertinent
- Social history: Non-smoking, no recreational drug use, or alcohol

Physical Exam

- Vital signs
  - Heart rate: 105 beats/minute
  - Blood pressure: 136/92 mmHg
  - Respiratory rate: 26 breaths/minute
  - Temperature: 100.0 °F
  - Oxygen saturation: 98% on room air
- General appearance: Alert, non-toxic appearing, no acute distress
- HEENT: No thyromegaly, no jugular venous distention
- Heart: Tachycardic rate and normal rhythm, no murmurs, no peripheral edema
- Lungs: Respirations non-labored, no wheezing, scant rales to the left lower lung fields
- Abdominal/GI: No abdominal distention, generalized abdominal tenderness but increased localized tenderness to palpation in the left upper quadrant, negative Murphy's sign, no guarding or rebound tenderness, no organomegaly, no costo-vertebral angle tenderness
- Genitourinary: Normal external female genitalia without lesions, swelling, masses, or tenderness. Normal vaginal mucosa. Scant white discharge in vaginal vault. Cervix nontender without lesions or erosions. Uterus is nontender but enlarged, approximately the size of a 12-week gestation. Adnexa without tenderness or palpable masses.
- Extremities: Non-edematous, no cyanosis or clubbing
- Back: No midline tenderness, pain reproduced on the left flank when lying flat from upright position
- Neuro: Alert, oriented, cranial nerves II-XII grossly intact, sensation and motor function of extremities equal and grossly intact
- Skin: No rashes or lesions
- Psych: Appropriate affect, cooperative

Pertinent Diagnostic Tests (Figs. 3.1, 3.2 and 3.3, Tables 3.1, 3.2, 3.3, 3.4, 3.5, 3.6 and 3.7)

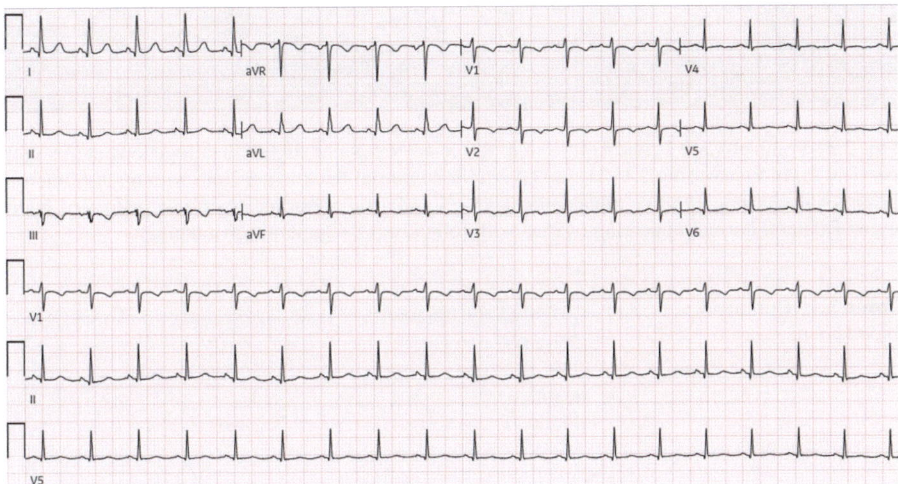

Fig. 3.1 Electrocardiogram (ECG): Sinus tachycardia with chronic T-wave inversions in III, aVF. (O. Clement's own image)

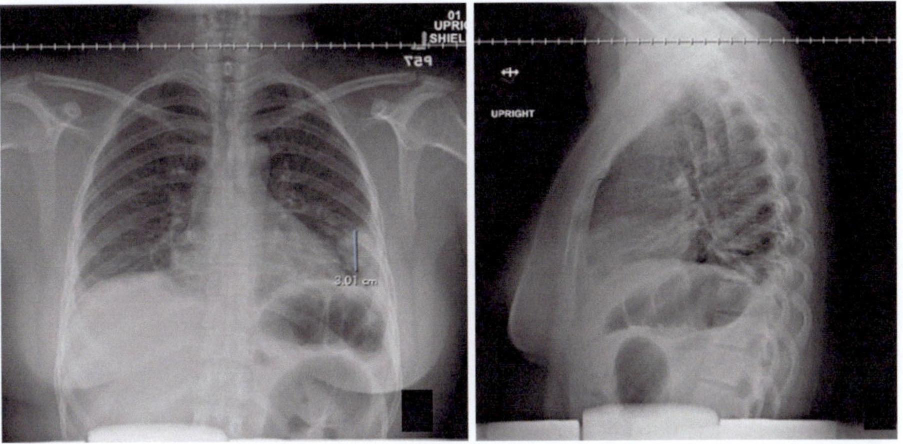

Fig. 3.2 Chest radiograph (CXR) posteroanterior(A) and lateral (B): Increased consolidative opacity in the periphery of the left lower lung and stable patchy basilar opacities in the lower lungs. Trace left pleural effusion. (O. Clement's own image)

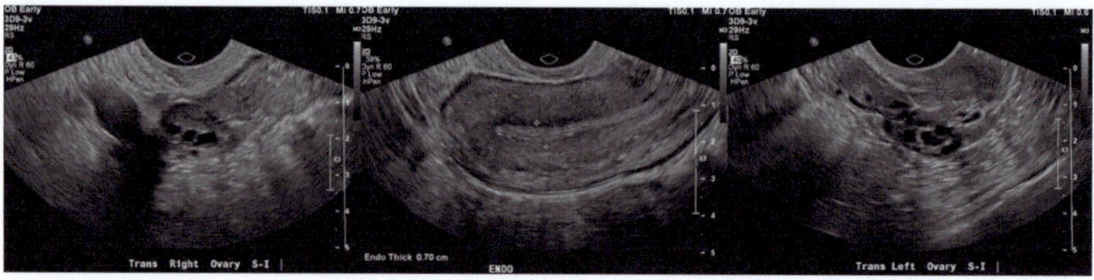

Fig. 3.3 Point-of-Care Pelvic Ultrasound: 8.9 × 4.3 × 5.8 cm slightly heterogenous uterus with cervical fibroid measuring 2.1 × 1.5 × 2.4 cm. Endometrial thickness 0.7 cm with no in-trauterine gestational sac, no definitive molar pregnancy. No adnexal abnormality or enlarged theca lutein cysts. Bilateral normal-appearing ovaries with follicles. (O. Clement's own image)

Table 3.1 Complete blood count

Complete blood count	
White blood cells	9.3×10^9/L
Hemoglobin	13.3 g/dL
Hematocrit	0.39
Platelets	391×10^9/L

Table 3.2 Comprehensive metabolic panel

Comprehensive metabolic panel	
Sodium	136 mEq/L
Potassium	4.1 mEq/L
Chloride	102 mEq/L
Bicarbonate	28 mEq/L
Glucose	98 mg/dL
Blood urea nitrogen (BUN)	7 mg/dL
Creatinine	0.49 mg/dL
Calcium	9.1 mg/dL
Total bilirubin	0.4 mg/dL
Alkaline phosphatase	113 units/L
Aspartate aminotransferase (AST)	21 units/L
Alanine aminotransferase (ALT)	22 units/L
Albumin	4.2 g/dL
Total protein	7.1 g/dL

Table 3.3 β-human chorionic gonadotropin (β-hCG)

β-hCG	136,629 mIU/mL

Table 3.4 Coagulopathy panel

Coagulopathy panel	
International normalized ratio (INR)	1.05
Prothrombin time (PT)	11.8 seconds
Activated partial thromboplastin time (aPTT)	27.1 seconds
D-Dimer	2.76 µg/mL Fibrinogen-Equivalent Units (FEU) (Reference range 0–0.50 µg/mL FEU)
Fibrinogen	290 mg/dL

Table 3.5 Blood type

Blood type	
ABO type	AB
Rh(D) antigen	+

Table 3.6 Thyroid panel

Thyroid-stimulating hormone (TSH)	2.3 µU/mL
Free T4	1.2 ng/dL

Table 3.7 Urinalysis

Urinalysis	
Color	Yellow
Appearance	Marked turbidity
Specific gravity	1.015
pH	6.0
Glucose	Negative
Bilirubin	Negative
Ketones	80
Protein	0
Leukocyte esterase	3+
Nitrites	Negative
White blood cells (WBCs)	9 WBCs/High-power field (HPF)
Red blood cells (RBCs)	8 RBCs/HPF
Squamous epithelial cells	Many Cells/HPF

Learning Points

Background

Gestational trophoblastic disease (GTD) is an overarching term, inclusive of all conditions in which there is abnormal proliferation of the placental trophoblast (Fig. 3.4). Diagnoses of various GTDs are made in patients of all reproductive ages but are more readily identified in women older than 45 years. The highest incidence occurs in Asian populations and Asian descendants [1].

A hydatidiform mole (i.e., a "molar pregnancy," which may be either partial hydatidiform or complete hydatidiform) is a type of GTD that originates from the fetal tissue, not the maternal tissue. Complete and partial hydatidiform moles are premalignant subtypes of GTD that are typically benign. Gestational trophoblastic neoplasia (GTN), however, is composed of malignant conditions, including invasive moles, choriocarcinoma, placental site trophoblastic tumors, and epithelioid trophoblastic tumors, which typically are invasive or may even metastasize. These trophoblastic tumors result from abnormal secretion of human chorionic gonadotropin (hCG), a hormone that is a key marker in the diagnosis of GTN and GTDs in general.

While GTN can result after molar pregnancy (Fig. 3.5), it may also result after a term/preterm pregnancy, abortion, or ectopic pregnancy. The incidence of GTN after complete molar pregnancy in the United States is reportedly between 18% and 29% [2]. The risk of subsequently developing an invasive mole is higher for patients

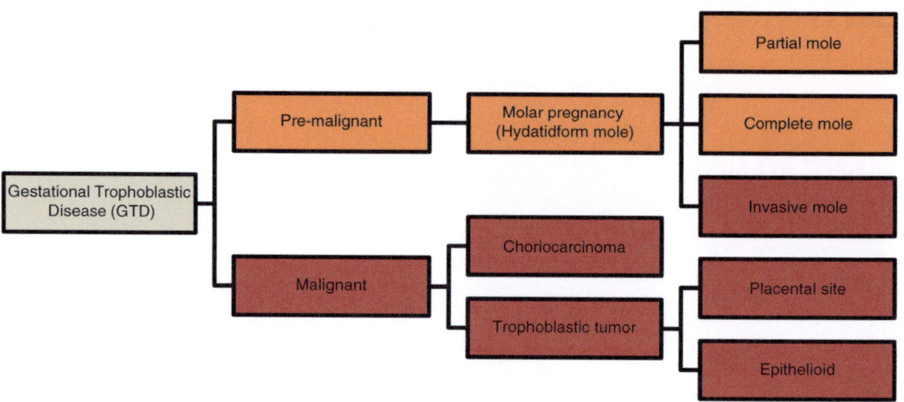

Fig. 3.4 General categories of gestational trophoblastic disease

with a history of a complete hydatidiform mole compared to those with a partial hydatidiform mole (15–20% vs. 0.5–1%, respectively) [1].

GTN is classified as either metastatic or non-metastatic based on its potential to produce highly vascular tumors that metastasize through the bloodstream. The lung and vagina are the two most common sites of metastasis while the brain and liver are less common sites of metastasis. Patients may rarely present with findings consistent with choriocarcinoma of another primary subtype: gastric, ovarian, or pulmonary, which have differing clinical courses and often worse prognoses [1].

The structure of hCG is composed of an alpha and a beta subunit. The alpha subunit is not a unique structure in the human body; rather, it is identical to that of several other hormones: thyroid-stimulating hormone (TSH), luteinizing hormone (LH), and follicle-stimulating hormone. The presence of elevated hCG (and therefore alpha subunits) leaves patients susceptible to concomitantly developing ovarian theca lutein cysts, hyperemesis gravidarum, preeclampsia, and thyroid storm, which can occur at hCG levels >100,000 mIU/mL. The beta subunit, however, is unique to hCG. Therefore, when performing laboratory testing, assays identify the beta subunit as a specific surrogate for the hCG protein. As a result, most persons in clinical medicine generally use the terms "hCG" and "β-hCG" interchangeably, though hCG more aptly refers to the hormone and β-hCG more aptly refers to the *measurement* of that same hormone.

Differential Diagnosis Early/unseen intrauterine pregnancy, early/unseen ectopic pregnancy, spontaneous abortion, germ cell tumors (germinoma, teratoma, embryonal carcinoma, yolk sac tumor, choriocarcinoma), pituitary production of hCG, preeclampsia, hyperthyroidism, and multiple fetuses.

Fig. 3.5 Hydatidiform molar pregnancy compared to normal pregnancy

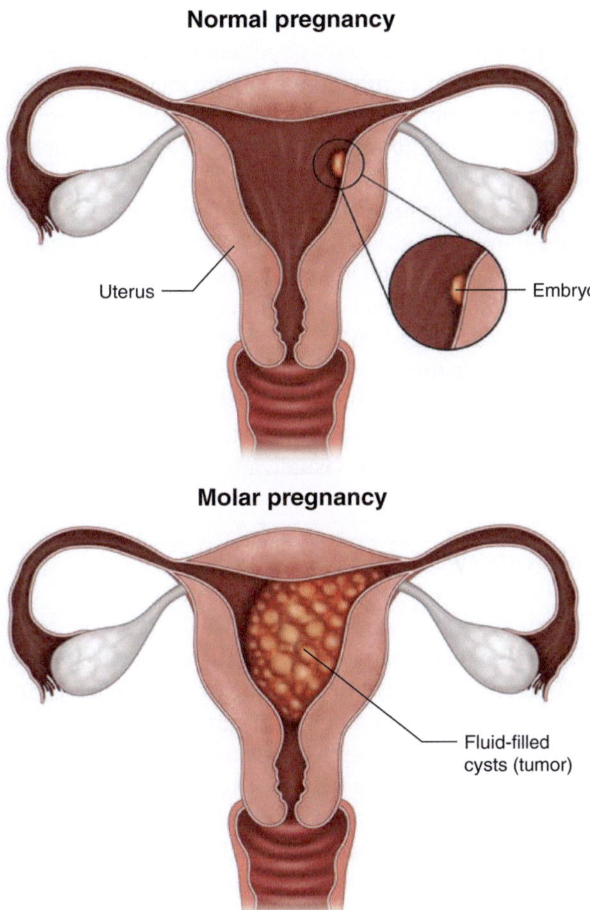

History and Physical Exam

The most common presenting symptom for a molar pregnancy is abnormal vaginal bleeding, which tends to occur during the first trimester. Some have described the blood as having a uniquely "prune juice" appearance. Another presenting complaint may be that of severe nausea and vomiting (hyperemesis) in the first trimester, which can be directly attributed to the abnormally high circulating levels of hCG. Occasionally, a patient may complain of passage of "grape-like" abnormal tissue from the vagina—again, typically in the first trimester. Other presenting complaints later in the first trimester or early second trimester may be more consistent with hyperthyroidism (nervousness, tremors, palpitations, insomnia, and weight loss). A patient may also present concerned for elevated blood pressure.

A history should elicit the details of the patient's complaint but also inquire regarding the patient's medical history. The most significant finding to suggest a molar pregnancy is a prior history of any type of molar or trophoblastic disease. Furthermore, for patients experiencing amenorrhea or ongoing vaginal bleeding 4–6 weeks after termination of pregnancy, evacuation of a nonviable pregnancy, or spontaneous abortion, consideration must be made for the diagnosis of GTD as opposed to retained products of conception, which is a far more common diagnosis [1].

Physical examination should obtain a full set of vital signs. The general physical exam should search for signs of hypertensive emergency, thyroid emergency, metastatic disease, and anemia. The more specific physical exam evaluation for GTD rests in the abdominal and genitourinary exam. The size of the uterus should be estimated by palpation of the abdomen externally and by bimanual exam. In more than 50% of patients with a complete mole, there is a larger uterus than expected for gestational age. Patients with an incomplete mole may have an intrauterine size similar to or smaller than expected for gestational age. Any vaginal bleeding or masses on palpation or visualization with a vaginal speculum should be noted.

Laboratory Studies

Important tests to obtain when there is a suspicion for GTD include a complete blood count and coagulation profile to evaluate for anemia, thrombocytopenia, disseminated intravascular coagulopathy, or other coagulopathy; a basic metabolic panel to evaluate for renal insufficiency or electrolyte disturbance; and a thyroid panel to screen for hyperthyroid emergency. Each patient should also have an evaluation for blood type and Rh type to appropriately transfuse blood if needed, and to receive anti-D immunoglobulin if the patient is Rh(D) negative.

Every patient with suspected GTD should have a quantitative serum β-hCG level measured. Human chorionic gonadotropin is a hormone produced by the placenta, meant to foster a fertilized and implanted egg at the uterine wall. It can typically be detected in a very predictable fashion in a normal pregnancy. About 11 days after conception, a serum β-hCG is usually detectable. About 2 weeks after conception, β-hCG can typically be detected by urine test (a qualitative study). Generally, serum β-hCG levels will double about every 72 hours, peaking at about 8–11 weeks and then gradually declining. In the diagnosis of GTD, the serum quantitative β-hCG level is often elevated (>100,000 mIU/mL), with the value often correlating with the disease burden. There are indeed two quite rare subsets of trophoblastic tumors (placental site trophoblastic tumors and epithelioid trophoblastic tumors) that secrete very low levels of β-hCG. An important use of the β-hCG value is to measure the rate at which the level is rising. This will help differentiate GTD from a missed abortion, a blighted ovum, or retained products of conception, depending on the context [1].

In the year 2000, the International Federation of Gynecology and Obstetrics revised established guidelines to assist in diagnosing a persistent tumor after molar pregnancy. These guidelines involve four different measures [3]:

1. β-hCG level that plateaus over a period of at least 3 weeks in 4 measurements (days 1, 7, 14, 21),
2. Increase in β-hCG level of 10% or more in 3 or more weekly measurements or over a period of at least 2 weeks (days 1, 7, 14).
3. β-hCG level remains elevated for 6 months or more,
4. Histological diagnosis of choriocarcinoma.

Imaging Findings

The widespread availability of ultrasound has contributed substantially to the early detection of GTD and it is the choice imaging modality for diagnosis of GTD. Routine first-trimester ultrasounds have significantly promoted early identification of GTD prior to the development of clinical symptoms.

Ultrasound features of complete hydatidiform moles are the following: absence of a fetus, no amniotic fluid, and an enlarged uterus that is filled with an echogenic mass with heterogenous hypoechoic cystic foci (classically referred to as "snowstorm" pattern) (Fig. 3.6). The term "cluster of grapes" was coined from the appearance of hydropic villi that comprise the cystic spaces. Additional findings include increased ovarian theca lutein cysts as a sequalae of increased β-hCG.

Partial hydatidiform moles may contain amorphous fetal parts or a nonviable fetus with less amniotic fluid than expected relative to the size of the uterus. There may also be cystic spaces that are "Swiss cheese" in appearance. For partial hydatidiform moles, the ratio of transverse diameter to anteroposterior diameter is >1.5, giving a more ovoid appearance compared to a complete mole. A rare alternative diagnosis can even be a molar pregnancy *with* a viable fetus, a type of twin pregnancy.

Imaging after diagnosis of a molar pregnancy, or in patients suspected of having GTN after a non-molar pregnancy, requires more advanced and often systemic imaging. Emergency imaging should be limited to detecting what is making a patient symptomatic. Chest radiography will look for metastatic disease (lesions >6 mm will often be visible). However, radiography is limited in identifying details of abnormalities when GTN is suspected. Therefore, most patients with abnormal

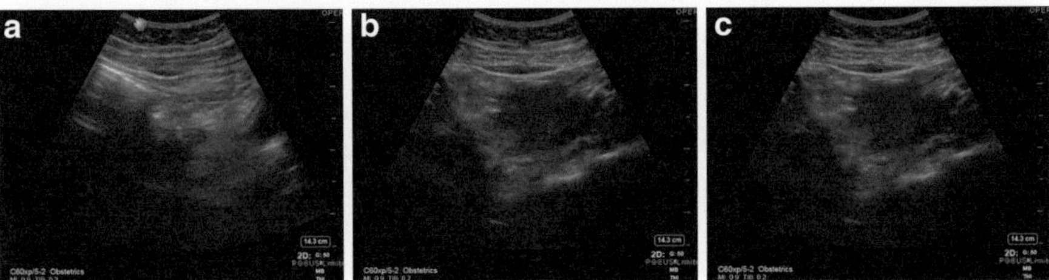

Fig. 3.6 Pelvic Ultrasound (**a**) Long uterus view (**b**) Short uterus view, (**c**) Transvaginal view: Enlarged uterus without a definitive intrauterine pregnancy. Abnormal appearing intrauterine contents. (Images courtesy of C. Bakunas, MD and R. Bower, MD)

findings on chest radiography will benefit from computed tomography (CT) of the chest and abdomen with arterial phase imaging through the liver for a more thorough evaluation of the disease process. In addition, when there are abnormal findings on the chest radiograph, magnetic resonance imaging (MRI) of the brain with contrast will typically eventually be performed to evaluate for brain metastases.

Management

Emergency department care of a patient with GTD should be focused on diagnosis and clinical stabilization of the patient. A patient presenting with respiratory distress due to metastatic disease or pulmonary edema may require endotracheal intubation and ventilation or non-invasive positive pressure ventilation. A patient with significant hemorrhage or coagulopathy should receive appropriate blood products and clotting elements. If seizure activity was described or witnessed, concern for eclampsia should manage seizures with benzodiazepines and high-dose magnesium and antihypertensives (hydralazine, labetalol) as needed for hypertension. If a patient demonstrates symptomatic hyperthyroidism, management should be expectant as per other populations with hyperthyroid disease (beta-blockers, thionamides, potassium iodide, and corticosteroids as indicated). Patients who are Rh(D) negative should receive anti-D immunoglobulin in protection of any future viable pregnancies.

After emergency stabilization, a patient with a molar pregnancy will ultimately require dilation and curettage (D&C) to evacuate the diseased tissue, or a hysterectomy with the same goal for women who are having severe hemorrhage or who do not have interest in further childbearing [1]. Of note, hysterectomy reduces but does not eliminate the risk of subsequent metastatic disease [1] (Fig. 3.6).

Management of a molar pregnancy after evacuation necessitates serial measurement of β-hCG levels to ensure remission, typically performed on a weekly basis until β-hCG becomes undetectable (<5 mIU/mL) for three weeks. Afterwards, patients are again tested monthly for six more months. Because of the intense surveillance necessary to detect malignant or recurrent disease, it is typically recommended that the patient does not get pregnant during any period of β-hCG surveillance. The healthcare team should facilitate reliable contraception.

The targeted diagnosis of GTN is not in the scope of emergency patient care. Patients with invasive moles or choriocarcinoma are staged by invasiveness of disease according to the International Federation of Gynecology and Obstetrics (FIGO) staging of GTN and are then considered low or high risk based on FIGO's adaptation of World Health Organization (WHO) prognostic scoring (0–12) [4]. Low-risk patients (scoring 0–6) are offered single-agent chemotherapy or hysterectomy, while high-risk patients (scoring $\geq$7) are offered multi-agent chemotherapy. Chemotherapy treats both metastatic and non-metastatic GTN, with a cure rate ranging between 80% and 100% depending on extent and subtype of disease [2]. Nevertheless, patients scoring $\geq$12 are considered ultra-high risk for complications including death and require specialized treatment with access to multidisciplinary teams, including interventional radiology, thoracic surgery, neurosurgery, and intensive care.

Consultation Considerations

The gynecology team should be consulted for any patient with a suspected hydatidiform mole for operative intervention by D&C or hysterectomy. A gynecologist will also navigate the appropriate diagnosis and management of the patient both in the hospital and in the outpatient setting.

Patients with suspected GTN should be referred to an oncology service, specifically a gynecology/oncology service, for admission for staging and appropriate interventions.

A pathologist, specifically a gynecologic pathologist, should be consulted if a patient has expelled products of conception that appear abnormal, as these products should be examined histologically to aid in accurate diagnosis of the patient's condition.

Emergency Department Course and Outcome

The emergency physician consulted a gynecology/oncology specialist with concern for GTN in this patient, who was then admitted to the specialty service. She underwent repeat CT imaging of the chest, abdomen, and pelvis, in addition to a CT of her brain. This demonstrated two pulmonary lesions (1 cm and 3 cm), pulmonary hemorrhage, and bilateral subsegmental pulmonary embolisms. These findings were attributed to metastatic disease. She was ultimately diagnosed with FIGO Stage 3 (WHO Score: 10) GTN. She was initiated on chemotherapy the next day: etoposide, methotrexate, and dactinomycin, alternating weekly with cyclophosphamide and vincristine (EMA-CO regimen) [1] and monitored for tumor lysis syndrome. Her hemoglobin was monitored inpatient, and cardiothoracic surgery was consulted on standby, following her case in anticipation of massive pulmonary hemorrhage resultant of initiation of chemotherapy. The patient was started on oral contraceptives, and her serum β-hCG was evaluated weekly while she was inpatient.

Key Points

- The greatest risk factor for gestational trophoblastic disease (GTD) is the prior history of GTD.
- A serum β-hCG level > 100,000 mIU/mL that is discordant with pregnancy dates and an abnormal pelvic ultrasound should be concerning for GTD.
- The vagina and lung are the most common regions of metastasis for gestational trophoblastic neoplasia. Due to their highly vascularized composition, lesions are high risk for acute hemorrhage.
- GTD can manifest as many other emergency conditions including hypertensive emergency, thyroid emergencies, preeclampsia and eclampsia, vaginal hemorrhage, altered mental status, or respiratory distress.

References

1. Eiriksson L, Dean E, Sebastianelli A, Salvador S, Comeau R, Jang JH, Bouchard-Fortier G, Osborne R, Sauthier P. Guideline no. 408: management of gestational trophoblastic diseases. J Obstet Gynaecol Can. 2021;43(1):91–105.e1. https://doi.org/10.1016/j.jogc.2020.03.001.
2. Berkowitz RS, Goldstein DP. Molar pregnancy. N Engl J Med. 2009;360(16):1639–45. https://doi.org/10.1056/NEJMcp0900696.
3. FIGO Oncology Committee. FIGO staging for gestational trophoblastic neoplasia 2000. Int J Gynaecol Obstet. 2002;77(3):285–7. https://doi.org/10.1016/s0020-7292(02)00063-2.
4. FIGO Committee on Gynecologic Oncology. Current FIGO staging for cancer of the vagina, fallopian tube, ovary, and gestational trophoblastic neoplasia. Int J Gynaecol Obstet. 2009;105(1):3–4. https://doi.org/10.1016/j.ijgo.2008.12.015.

Spontaneous Abortion

Lost Ones

Cindy Amilcar

Case

A 37-year-old woman presents to the emergency department (ED) for vaginal bleeding ongoing the past 2 days. On average, the patient notes that she has been using two panty liners each day. She denies having seen any clots or anything that appears like bodily tissue. She reports a mild, intermittent bilateral lower abdominal/pelvic cramping. She rates her pain 2 out of 10. She denies fevers, dysuria, diarrhea, or vaginal discharge. Her last menstrual period was two months ago.

- Past medical history: None
- Past surgical history: None
- Medications: Prenatal vitamins
- Allergies: No known drug allergies
- Family history: Mother has hypertension
- Social history: Non-smoker. No alcohol use. No illicit drug use.

Physical Exam

- Vital signs:
  - Heart rate: 83 beats/minute
  - Blood pressure: 129/82 mmHg
  - Respiratory rate: 16 breaths/minute
  - Temperature: 99.1 °F

Supplementary Information The online version contains supplementary material available at https://doi.org/10.1007/978-3-031-70118-4_4.

C. Amilcar (✉)
Department of Emergency Medicine, McGovern School of Medicine, University of Texas Health Sciences Center at Houston, Houston, TX, USA

- Oxygen saturation: 98% on room air
- General appearance: Appears stated age, in no acute distress
- HEENT
  - Head: Normocephalic, atraumatic
  - Eyes: Pupils equal and reactive to light, conjunctiva moist and without pallor
- Heart: Regular rate and rhythm, equal pulses
- Lungs: Normal breath sounds, normal effort
- Abdominal/GI: Soft, non-distended, non-tender
- Genitourinary: Trace blood in the vaginal vault. Internal and external cervical os closed. No adnexal tenderness or cervical motion tenderness.
- Extremities: No edema, normal range of motion
- Neuro: Alert and oriented to person, place, and time. No focal deficits.
- Skin: Warm and dry

Pertinent Diagnostic Tests (Fig. 4.1, Tables 4.1, 4.2, 4.3, 4.4, 4.5 and 4.6)

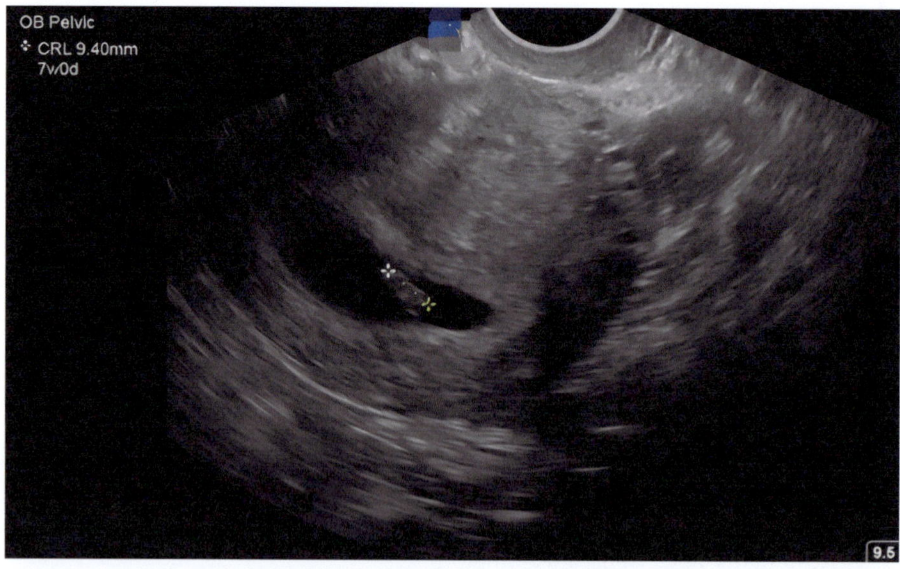

Fig. 4.1 Point-of-care pelvic ultrasound (POCUS): Live intrauterine pregnancy with fetal heart rate of 150 beats/minute. Estimated age by crown rump length is 7 weeks and 0 days. (Image courtesy of Carrie Bakunas, MD.)

Table 4.1 Complete blood count

Complete blood count	
White blood cells	13.8×10^9/L
Hemoglobin	12.7 g/dL
Hematocrit	39.7%
Platelets	346×10^9/μL

Table 4.2 Basic metabolic panel

Basic metabolic panel	
Sodium	135 mEq/L
Potassium	4.1 mEq/L
Chloride	103 mEq/L
Bicarbonate	23 mEq/L
Glucose	94 mg/dL
Blood urea nitrogen (BUN)	9 mg/dL
Creatinine	0.6 mg/dL
Calcium	9.2 mg/dL

Table 4.3 Coagulopathy panel

Coagulopathy panel	
International normalized ratio (INR)	1.1
Prothrombin time (PT)	12.6 seconds
Activated partial thromboplastin time (aPTT)	26.7 seconds

Table 4.4 Urinalysis

Urinalysis	
Color	Yellow
Appearance	Clear
Specific gravity	1.011
pH	7.0
Glucose	Negative
Bilirubin	Negative
Ketones	1+
Protein	Negative
Leukocyte esterase	Negative
Nitrites	Negative
White blood cells (WBC)	2 WBCs/high-power field (HPF)
Red blood cells (RBC)	10 RBCs/HPF
Squamous epithelial cells	0–5 cells/HPF

Table 4.5 Type and screen

Type and screen	
ABO/RH	O Positive

Table 4.6 Beta human chorionic gonadotropin

Beta human chorionic gonadotropin	211,467 mIU/mL

Learning Points

Background

Spontaneous abortion is defined as the unplanned loss of a nonviable intrauterine pregnancy prior to 20 weeks' gestation. "Spontaneous abortion" and "early pregnancy loss" are terms often used interchangeably [1]. *Early pregnancy loss* specifically refers to the miscarriage of a pregnancy in the first trimester (up to 12 weeks and 6 days) [2]. The categories of spontaneous abortions include threatened, inevitable, incomplete,

complete, missed, and septic (Table 4.7, Fig. 4.2). Approximately 30% of all pregnancies will have an episode of vaginal bleeding during the first 20 weeks of gestation. Fifty percent of those episodes will result in a spontaneous abortion [1].

Fetal chromosome abnormalities account for greater than half of all spontaneous abortions [2]. Advanced maternal age and previous spontaneous abortions are the most notable risk factors for a chromosomal abnormality. Women 20–30 years old experience early pregnancy loss with a frequency of 9–17%. This frequency increases to 40% for women 40 years of age or older [2].

Other risk factors for spontaneous abortions include tobacco, alcohol, and illicit drug use, uterine anatomical abnormalities, and maternal infection.

Spontaneous abortions account for more than 900,000 emergency department visits annually in the United States [3].

Differential Diagnosis ectopic pregnancy, subchorionic hematoma, molar pregnancy, implantation bleeding, fibroids, cervical or vaginal trauma.

History and Physical Exam

The diagnosis of a spontaneous abortion is based on history and physical exam. A thorough history should question [4]:

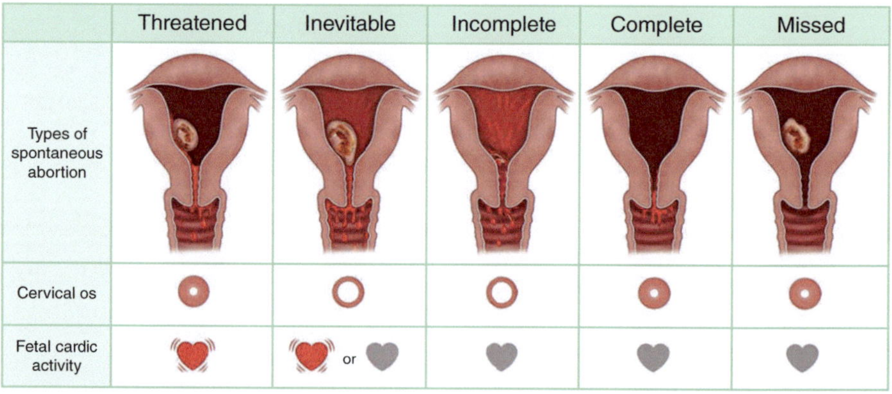

Fig. 4.2 Categories of spontaneous abortion

Table 4.7 Categories of spontaneous abortion

Types of abortion	Status of cervical Os	Fetal tissue passage
Threatened	Closed	No
Inevitable	Open	No
Incomplete	Open	Some
Complete	Closed	Yes
Missed	Closed	No
Septic[a]	Open	No or some

[a]*Septic abortion* is characterized by any retained products of conception resulting in infection within the uterus as a complication

1. Last menstrual period
2. Obstetric history (i.e., parity, prenatal care, previous pregnancies)
3. Presence of abdominal/pelvic cramping or pain
4. Vaginal bleeding (i.e., duration, quantity of sanitary napkins used, passage of clots)

The physical exam should begin with an assessment of the vital signs. Patients should be triaged as stable or unstable based on vital signs reflecting rapid or voluminous blood loss or sepsis. It is important to note that patients in the late stages of their first trimester have an increase in blood volume and subsequently can lose a substantial amount of blood before vital signs become abnormal [4]. A fever can be a sign of a septic abortion, a urinary tract infection, a sexually transmitted infection, or other infection which may increase the likelihood of a spontaneous abortion.

The pelvic exam is necessary to categorize the type of spontaneous abortion. A speculum will allow for visualization of the external cervical os and vaginal vault for identification of any bleeding, discharge, products of conception, or lesions. A bimanual exam will determine whether the internal cervical os is open or closed. An open cervical os in the first trimester can indicate an inevitable or an incomplete spontaneous abortion. If one fingertip fits through the os, it is considered open about 1 cm. If two fingertips fit through the os, it is estimated open about 2 cm. A bimanual exam may also identify any tenderness or masses at the ovaries, fallopian tubes, uterus, or cervix.

Laboratory Studies

The diagnosis of spontaneous abortion is clinical, but there are some laboratory values that are important to document for guiding management. A complete blood count (CBC) will evaluate for anemia which may reflect the rate and volume of vaginal bleeding. An elevation in the white blood cell count (WBC) can indicate an infection. However, the WBC can naturally be elevated in pregnancy and should be used in conjunction with a total clinical evaluation if concerned about an infection.

The patient's blood type and rhesus factor (Rh) should be obtained in case the patient needs a blood transfusion. Moreover, a patient who is Rh negative should receive $Rh_o(D)$ immune globulin to prevent RhD isoimmunization, which is protective for any potential future pregnancies.

Urinalysis should be used to evaluate for a urinary tract infection. Even if the patient may lack typical symptoms (e.g., dysuria or frequency), asymptomatic bacteriuria, when left untreated, can result in pyelonephritis in 30% of pregnancies [5].

Quantifying the serum beta human chorionic gonadotropin (hCG) can help determine whether the pregnancy is producing the expected hCG level for the gestational age. The hCG value can be repeated to determine if a trend is reassuring or concerning. With a normal pregnancy, hCG levels rise by about 50% every 2 days, but when there is early pregnancy failure, the hCG level declines by about 50% every 2 days [6].

Imaging Findings

An ultrasound (transvaginal or transabdominal) is one of the most important tests to determine the location of the pregnancy and whether the pregnancy is viable. A reassuring ultrasound or a threatened abortion will demonstrate an intrauterine pregnancy (IUP) with a normal fetal heart rate (Fig. 4.3). However, an abnormal ultrasound can identify other concerning diagnoses (e.g., ectopic pregnancy). A missed abortion would identify an intrauterine pregnancy without a reassuring fetal heart rate. An incomplete abortion would demonstrate retained products of conception in the uterus or cervix. An ultrasound of a completed abortion would show an empty uterus (Fig. 4.4).

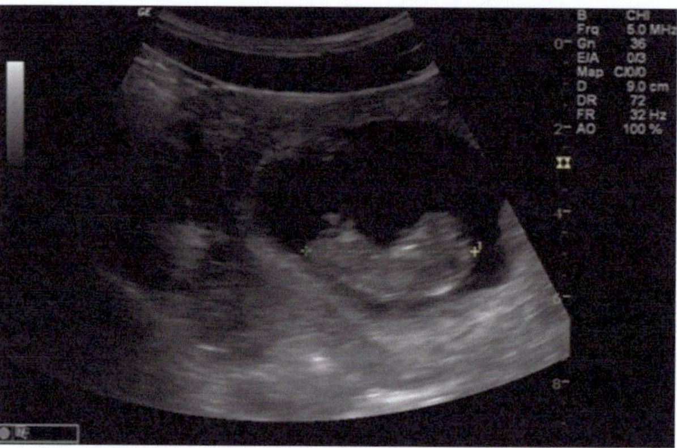

Fig. 4.3 Transabdominal Pelvic Ultrasound: Normal intrauterine pregnancy. (Images courtesy of C. Bakunas, MD and R. Bower, MD)

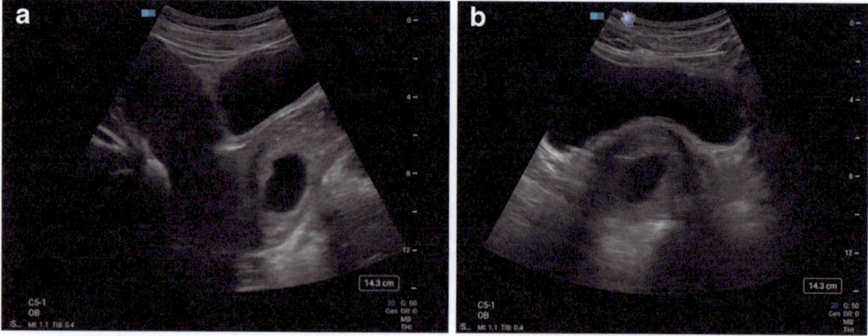

Fig. 4.4 Transabdominal Pelvic Ultrasound (**a**) Long uterus view, (**b**) Short uterus view: No confirmed intrauterine pregnancy. (Images courtesy of C. Bakunas, MD and R. Bower, MD)

Management

Treatment options for spontaneous abortions include expectant management, medical management, and surgical management. All options have been shown to be effective [2]. Unless there are any systemic medical complications requiring specific intervention, the management selected for a medically stable patient can often be based on patient preference or physician recommendation.

Expectant management refers to the natural expulsion of the fetus without any intervention. Most cases of uncomplicated spontaneous abortions are simply left to expectant management. Within 2 to 6 weeks, 80% to 90% of incomplete spontaneous abortions will be successfully eradicated without medical intervention and without increased rates of complications [7]. Missed abortions have a 65% to 75% completion rate in the same time frame when left to expectant management [7]. Patients choosing expectant management typically experience moderate-to-heavy bleeding and cramping until the products of conception are completely expelled in up to 2 to 6 weeks. These patients can typically be discharged with analgesia and strict return precautions regarding increasing volume of bleeding, worsening of pain, or systemic signs of illness. The patient should also be informed that surgical management may be needed if expectant management fails.

Pharmaceuticals may be offered to aid in expulsion of a failed pregnancy. This option is safe for patients without infection, hemorrhage, bleeding disorders, or severe anemia. Patients who want to shorten the natural course of expulsion are more likely to choose this medical management [2]. The current drug of choice is misoprostol 800 mcg prescribed vaginally, sublingually, or orally. Misoprostol is a prostaglandin E1 analogue which stimulates uterine contractions and cervical ripening to aid in excretion of the products of conception. A second dose can be given if the desired outcome does not occur within 7 days after the first dose [2]. Another approach is to utilize mifepristone, which has restricted distribution in the United States. If available, mifepristone 200 mg can be given orally 24 hours before misoprostol. Mifepristone is a progesterone receptor inhibitor which antagonizes the endometrium and myometrium. The combination of mifepristone-misoprostol is significantly more effective than misoprostol alone and decreases the need for surgical intervention due to failed medical management [8]. As in expectant management, patients should utilize analgesia for the expected discomfort associated when using pharmaceutical agents. They should be educated on the expected course of bleeding and cramping when taking these medications. Patients should understand that if medical management fails, surgical intervention may be necessary.

Completed abortion or successful completion of expulsion of products of conception from an unviable pregnancy is usually associated with the patient experiencing symptomatic relief (i.e., hemostasis, relief of pain) along with serum β-hCG levels approaching zero [2]. If a confirmatory ultrasound is to be performed, it is usually done after 1 to 2 weeks to confirm an emptied uterus [2].

Surgical management is typically performed by dilation of the os and manual curettage of the uterus (dilation & curettage, D&C), removing the products of conception performed by a person skilled in the procedure, usually in the operating room as a sterile procedure. Although a patient can request surgical intervention upon diagnosis of spontaneous abortion, it is normally reserved for patients who are hemodynamically unstable, have active hemorrhage, infection, bleeding disorders, or other concerning medical comorbidities [2]. Surgical management offers an immediate completion of a spontaneous abortion compared to the prolonged approaches of using medications or expectant management, often simplifying the outpatient course.

A septic abortion is a failed intrauterine pregnancy complicated by a pelvic infection. It can occur due to ascending sexually transmitted disease, unaddressed retained products of conception, or from attempted pregnancy intervention using non-sterile instruments. The infection is typically polymicrobial. Overall worldwide mortality is 20–50%. The patient will often have systemic signs (e.g., fever), nausea/vomiting, and tachycardia in addition to vaginal bleeding or discharge with abdominal/pelvic pain. If the case is of a suspected septic abortion, blood cultures should also be ideally obtained prior to providing any indicated fluids or vasopressors for management of sepsis and broad-spectrum intravenous antibiotics (IV): ampicillin, gentamicin, clindamycin (or metronidazole). Computed tomography of the abdomen/pelvis with IV contrast may be needed to evaluate for the extent of tissue damage. A tetanus booster vaccination should also be considered.

Regardless of the management selected, an Rh-negative patient should receive $Rh_o(D)$ immune globulin within 72 hours of the onset of spontaneous abortion or when vaginal bleeding was noted [9]. Although the risk of alloimmunization is low, the consequences for a potential future pregnancy could be quite serious if this prophylaxis is not taken.

Consultation Considerations

The gynecology team should be consulted promptly for all hemodynamically unstable vaginal hemorrhages in pregnancy because despite emergency interventions undertaken in the emergency setting, these patients could ultimately require surgical intervention to achieve hemostasis.

Options for medical management or surgical management for spontaneous abortions are subject to local customs and legislation. An obstetric or gynecologist consultant may be more familiar with recommendations on local options compared to an emergency specialist.

A septic abortion will require admission to the hospital for IV antibiotics. These patients will also require a D&C or more extensive surgical intervention to remove remaining products of conception, any devastated tissue, or any abscesses.

Most patients experiencing uncomplicated spontaneous abortions can be managed in the outpatient setting with gynecology clinic follow-up. Many patients who desired the pregnancy may now be experiencing an unexpected sense of loss. These patients should be comforted as any other person suddenly experiencing loss in the emergency setting. The patients should be made aware that *most* cases of spontaneous abortion are not resultant of any decisions or actions for which the patient had control. Furthermore, the experience of a spontaneous abortion in itself does not negate the potential for a successful future pregnancy. Mental health consultations should be made as necessary.

Emergency Department Course and Outcome

The patient was ultimately diagnosed with a threatened abortion based on the history of vaginal bleeding, closed internal cervical os, and viable IUP on ultrasound. There was no evidence of heavy bleeding, significant anemia, or hemodynamic instability to suggest the need for admission or other intervention. The patient was found to be Rh positive and did not require $Rh_o(D)$ immune globulin. She did not require any medical intervention. Return precautions, including (but not limited to) syncope, increased vaginal bleeding, and worsening abdominal pain, were discussed with her. She was discharged to her home and encouraged to see her obstetrician in clinic in 2 days for a reassessment.

Key Points

- Spontaneous abortion is defined as unanticipated pregnancy loss at less than 20 weeks' gestation.
- There are several types of spontaneous abortion differentiated by history and pelvic exam with ultrasound.
- There are three treatment options when a pregnancy is no longer viable: expectant, medical, or surgical.
- $Rh_o(D)$ immune globulin should be given as prophylaxis within 72 hours of beginning of symptoms to any patient experiencing a spontaneous abortion, to decrease risk of alloimmunization.

References

1. Dulay A. Spontaneous abortion. In: Abnormalities of pregnancy. Merck Manual; 2022.
2. American College of Obstetricians and Gynecologists' Committee on Practice Bulletins—Gynecology. ACOG practice bulletin no. 200: early pregnancy loss. Obstet Gynecol. 2018;132(5):e197–207. https://doi.org/10.1097/AOG.0000000000002899.
3. Benson LS, Magnusson SL, Gray KE, Quinley K, Kessler L, Callegari LS. Early pregnancy loss in the emergency department, 2006-2016. J Am Coll Emerg Phys Open. 2021;2(6):e12549. https://doi.org/10.1002/emp2.12549.
4. Motola I, Panakos P. Abortion, spontaneous. In: 5-minute emergency consult. Unbound Medicine. 2016. http://emergency.unboundmedicine.com/emergency/view/5-Minute_Emergency_Consult/307234/all/Abortion__Spontaneous. Accessed 4 May 2023.
5. Smaill FM, Vazquez JC. Antibiotics for asymptomatic bacteriuria in pregnancy. Cochrane Database Syst Rev. 2019;2019(11):CD000490. https://doi.org/10.1002/14651858.CD000490.pub4.

6. Muleba N, Casey B, Wells E, Mcintire D, Leveno K. Human chronic gonadotropin levels following spontaneous abortion in the first trimester. Am J Obstet Gynecol. 2005;193(6 Suppl):S116. https://doi.org/10.1016/j.ajog.2005.10.409.
7. Butler C, Kelsberg G, St Anna L, Crawford P. Clinical inquiries. How long is expectant management safe in first-trimester miscarriage? J Fam Pract. 2005;54(10):889–90.
8. Ngoc NT, Blum J, Raghavan S, Nga NT, Dabash R, Diop A, Winikoff B. Comparing two early medical abortion regimens: mifepristone+misoprostol vs. misoprostol alone. Contraception. 2011;83(5):410–7. https://doi.org/10.1016/j.contraception.2010.09.002.
9. Alves C, Rapp A. Spontaneous abortion. In: StatPearls [internet]. StatPearls Publishing. 2022. https://www.ncbi.nlm.nih.gov/books/NBK560521/

Placenta Previa

Late Pregnancy Vaginal Bleeding—Oh No!

Sangeeta S. Sakaria

Case

A 39-year-old woman, G3P1 at 31 weeks gestation, presents with 4 hours of painless vaginal bleeding. She was sitting at her desk at work when the bleeding began suddenly. Since then, she has used 2 regular maxi pads in the last 4 hours. She has not had any cramping or leakage of fluids. She notes passing one quarter-sized clot when the bleeding began. There has not been any injury to her abdomen or pelvis that she recalls.

She has had routine prenatal care with her obstetrician who is located approximately one hour away from the receiving emergency department. As far as she understands, this pregnancy has been uncomplicated. The obstetrician mentioned that they would be "keeping an eye on" the position of her placenta, but that they did "not need to worry about it right now." The patient missed her last scheduled ultrasound appointment a few weeks ago because of childcare issues, and her next ultrasound is scheduled for next week.

The patient denies fever, chills, chest pain, difficulty breathing, urinary symptoms, or leg swelling. She notes that she had one day of spotting last week, but since

S. S. Sakaria (✉)
Department of Emergency Medicine, Cambridge Health Alliance, Cambridge, MA, USA
e-mail: ssakaria@challiance.org

A. A. Kosoko (ed.), *Emergency Medicine Case-Based Guide*,
https://doi.org/10.1007/978-3-031-70118-4_5

it resolved the same day, she did not think it warranted going in to see her obstetrician. She has appreciated regular fetal movements with no change in frequency of movement.

- Past medical history: First trimester miscarriage approximately one year ago
- Past surgical history: Appendectomy, cesarean section delivery with first child
- Medications: Prenatal vitamins, vitamin D
- Allergies: No known drug allergies
- Family history: Father with hypertension
- Social history: Former cigarette smoker at 2–3 cigarettes per day; quit prior to this pregnancy and prior pregnancies as well. Does not drink alcohol while pregnant and denies ever using recreational drugs.

Physical Exam

- Vital signs
  - Heart rate: 112 beats/minute
  - Blood pressure: 104/68 mmHg
  - Respiratory rate: 22 breaths/minute
  - Temperature: 37.3 °C
  - Oxygen saturation: 97% on room air
- General appearance: Appears stated age, no acute distress
- HEENT
  - Head: Atraumatic, normocephalic
  - Eyes: Pupils equal, round, and reactive to light (3–2 mm), external ocular movements are normal, normal conjunctiva—no pallor
- Heart: Tachycardia, regular rhythm, 2+ distal pulses in all extremities
- Lungs: Lungs clear to auscultation bilaterally, no increased work of breathing
- Abdominal/GI: Soft, nontender, bowel sounds present, gravid with fundus approximately 10 cm above the umbilicus
- Genitourinary: Normal external genitalia, bright red vaginal bleeding noted on a maxi pad, no clots noted, internal exam deferred
- Rectal: Deferred
- Extremities: Trace nonpitting edema to bilateral feet and ankles, no tenderness, no deformity, tolerates full range of motion
- Back: No step offs, no deformities
- Neuro: Alert, oriented, moving all extremities, 5/5 strength all extremities, sensation to light touch equal bilaterally, reflexes 2+
- Skin: Warm, well-perfused
- Psych: Normal mood, linear thought process

Pertinent Diagnostic Tests (Fig. 5.1, Tables 5.1, 5.2, 5.3, 5.4 and 5.5)

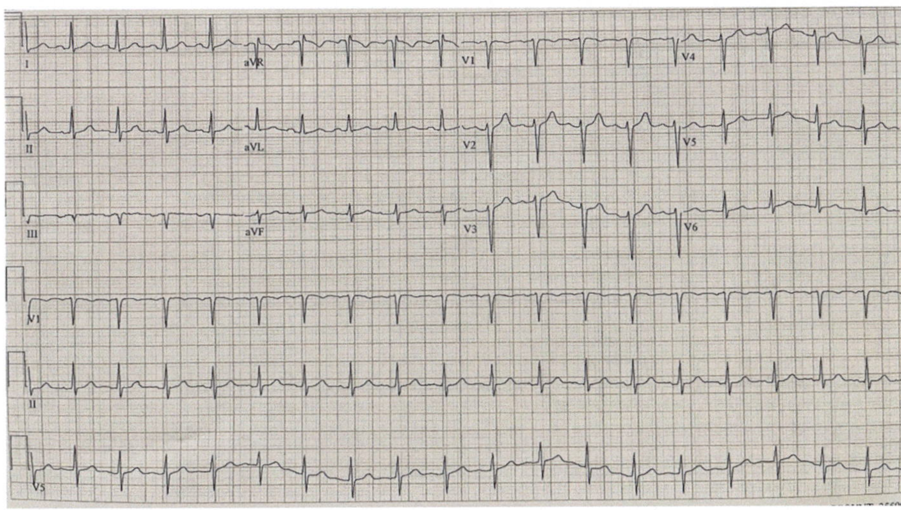

Fig. 5.1 Electrocardiogram (ECG): Sinus tachycardia. (Author's own image)

Table 5.1 Complete blood count

Complete blood count	
White blood cells	$7 \times 10^9/\mu L$
Hemoglobin	11 g/dL
Hematocrit	33%
Platelets	$246 \times 10^9/\mu L$

Table 5.2 Comprehensive metabolic panel

Comprehensive metabolic panel	
Sodium	135 mEq/L
Potassium	3.8 mEq/L
Chloride	104 mEq/L
Bicarbonate	24 mEq/L
Glucose	96 mg/dL
Blood urea nitrogen (BUN)	18 mg/dL
Creatinine	0.9 mg/dL
Calcium	8.4 mg/dL
Total bilirubin	0.8 mg/dL
Alkaline phosphatase	56 units/L
Aspartate aminotransferase (AST)	48 units/L
Alanine aminotransferase (ALT)	42 units/L
Albumin	3.2 g/dL
Total protein	6.8 g/dL

Table 5.3 Coagulopathy panel

Coagulopathy panel	
International normalized ratio (INR)	0.96
Prothrombin time (PT)	11.8 seconds
Activated partial thromboplastin time (aPTT)	24.2 seconds

Table 5.4 Blood type

Blood type	
ABO type	O
Rh(D) antigen	+

Table 5.5 Urinalysis (UA)

Urinalysis (UA)	
Color	Yellow
Appearance	Clear
Specific gravity	1.010
pH	7.0
Glucose	Negative
Bilirubin	Negative
Ketones	Negative
Protein	Negative
Leukocyte esterase	Negative
Nitrites	Negative
White blood cells (WBC)	2 WBCs/High-Power Field (HPF)
Red blood cells (RBC)	0 RBCs/HPF
Squamous epithelial cells	0–5 cells/HPF

Learning Points

Background

Placenta previa is an obstetric complication in which the placenta is approaching or overlying the internal cervical os. A normal placenta attaches to the superior portion of the uterus. Placenta previa can range from a low-lying placenta (attaching to the lower uterine segment within 2–3.5 cm of the internal os but does not reach it) to a complete (total) previa (completely covers the internal os) [1] (Fig. 5.2). The incidence of placenta previa is approximately 0.3–2% of pregnancies in the third trimester with cases increasing in recent years. Evidence has shown increasing cases of placenta previa correlating with increased rates of cesarean sections, increasing maternal age, and utilization of infertility treatments [2, 3].

The underlying cause of placenta previa is not well understood, but research studies have identified several independent risk factors: prior cesarean delivery, maternal age > 35 years, increased number of gestations and deliveries, prior pregnancy termination, intrauterine scarring, smoking, and infertility treatment [1]. The prevalence of placenta previa increases mid-pregnancy. Up to 85% of cases resolve prior to delivery and are inconsequential. Patients diagnosed with complete previa

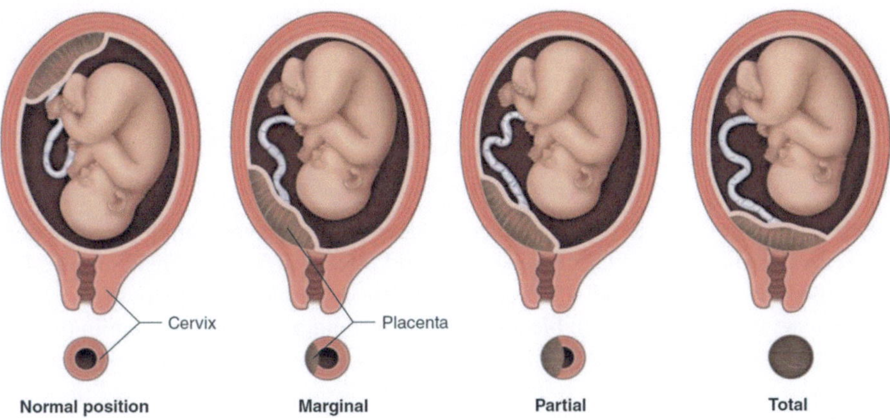

Fig. 5.2 Grades of placenta previa

mid-pregnancy are more likely to have the diagnosis persist into the third trimester compared to women with an incomplete previa mid-pregnancy.

Placenta previa is a major risk factor for maternal hemorrhage, which is one of the three leading causes of maternal death in the world [4, 5]. Specifically, placenta previa tends to cause poor maternal outcomes due to increased rates of sepsis, vasa previa, malpresentation, postpartum hemorrhage, and increased rates of peripartum hysterectomy. Diagnoses of placenta previa made in the emergency setting often lead to cesarean delivery to avoid the risk of hemorrhage that can be associated with vaginal delivery. Poor neonatal outcomes associated with placenta previa include APGAR scores <7 at both 1 and 5 minutes, lower birth weight, intrauterine growth retardation, congenital malformations, and increased neonatal mortality [6, 7].

Differential Diagnosis placenta accreta spectrum, placental abruption, uterine rupture, vaginal laceration, cervical laceration.

History and Physical Exam

Placenta previa often presents with a chief complaint of painless vaginal bleeding in the second or third trimester of pregnancy. A history should include any reports of pain and descriptions of the patterns of pain which could suggest labor or placental abruption. The estimated amount of blood loss is helpful to understand the severity of hemorrhage and may be best described by counting the number of soaked sanitary products used (see Table 5.6). Estimating total blood loss in this way, rather than relying solely on the physical exam findings, may improve clinical decision making.

Any prior episodes of vaginal bleeding should be noted because patients with placenta previa often have a sentinel bleed prior to more significant bleeding. Patients should be asked about any recent trauma to the abdomen or pelvis or even

Table 5.6 Estimated blood loss based on sanitary products used [8]

Sanitary product	Estimated blood loss if saturated
Tampons	20 mL to 34 mL
Pads (sanitary napkins)	31 mL to 52 mL
Period underwear	Up to 50 mL (can vary significantly by brand)

any penetrative sexual activity which could have prompted vaginal bleeding. A personal medical history and family history should inquire about propensity to bleed in other medical situations and whether there is history of bleeding diathesis.

Because most patients with bleeding from placenta previa will present in the latter portion of pregnancy, the prenatal course should be reviewed. The patient will often have already received a routine prenatal ultrasound which evaluated the fetus and the position of the placenta.

Assess for risk factors including smoking, infertility treatments, prior cesarean sections, or other uterine procedures that could cause intrauterine scarring, which would give the patient a higher risk of placenta previa.

The physical exam should focus on identifying any signs of hemodynamic instability due to hemorrhage. Vital signs should be repeated regularly in the emergency setting, and the physical exam should evaluate for signs of anemia or hypovolemia. Importantly, if placenta previa is considered as a cause for vaginal bleeding, an internal exam of the vagina (speculum exam, manual exam) should be deferred until the location of the placenta is confirmed by ultrasound. This can avoid unnecessary trauma to the cervical os, which could trigger critical vaginal bleeding. After confirming the location of the placenta, a carefully performed speculum exam can evaluate for other causes of bleeding, including cervical or vaginal lacerations.

Laboratory Studies

Laboratory studies do not aid in the diagnosis of placenta previa but are necessary for clinical management. A complete blood count (CBC) will particularly help to evaluate for anemia and for possible thrombocytopenia. A type and crossmatch including Rh (ABO type/Rh) should be prepared for possible blood transfusion. An activated partial thromboplastin time (aPTT), prothrombin time (PT), and international normalized ratio (INR) will assess for coagulopathy. If significant bleeding is reported or present on exam, serial hemoglobin and hematocrit levels should be ordered to trend values.

Imaging Findings

Ultrasound is the imaging modality of choice when evaluating a patient for placenta previa. Transvaginal ultrasound is safe to perform even with a known diagnosis of placenta previa and is the preferred ultrasound method [9]. It is highly specific and sensitive in diagnosing placenta previa, and antenatal diagnosis can help optimize obstetrical management [3, 6]. Transvaginal ultrasound is preferred to transabdominal ultrasound, especially in the third trimester, as the presenting fetal parts may obstruct the transabdominal view of the internal os.

If the placenta terminates within 2–3.5 cm of the internal cervical os, it is considered a low-lying placenta. If the placenta covers part of the internal cervix, it is defined as an incomplete previa. If the placenta completely covers the internal cervix, the patient has a complete (total) placenta previa. Patients who have had regular prenatal care will often have already had placenta previa or a low-lying placenta diagnosed in mid-pregnancy. It is common for a mid-pregnancy placenta previa to resolve as the placenta grows toward the fundus as gestation progresses. It is especially common for a placenta previa that is attached posteriorly to completely resolve spontaneously by the time of delivery [10].

If the ultrasound demonstrates that the placenta attaches anteriorly, the patient will be at increased risk for higher rate of prenatal bleeding, shorter gestational age, low birth weight, lower Apgar scores, increased risk of postpartum hemorrhage, longer hospitalizations, and higher rates of both transfusion and hysterectomy compared to posterior attachment. Placental attachment at a prior cesarean incision site significantly increases the incidence of a complete placenta previa [11].

If a placenta previa is identified on ultrasound, the imaging should also be reviewed for diagnoses in the placenta accreta spectrum. For patients >35 years old who have had two or more prior cesarean sections and have an anteriorly attached placenta previa, the incidence of a concomitant placenta accreta approaches 40% [12]. Placenta accreta occurs when the depth of the placenta extends into the myometrium or beyond, which can lead to life-threatening hemorrhage.

Management

The most important intervention in the emergency department is hemodynamic stabilization, as indicated. The patient should have reliable large-bore peripheral intravenous lines placed in case rapid transfusion of blood products becomes necessary. Transfusion of packed red blood cells or other blood products will depend on the degree of bleeding and the patient's hemodynamic status. If the patient is actively experiencing hemorrhage that is producing concerning signs of hypovolemia or anemia, transfusion of blood products should be started regardless of the initial hemoglobin or hematocrit level.

The well-being of the fetus should be evaluated by measuring fetal heart tones by Doppler ultrasound or point-of-care ultrasound. Preferably, the dynamic state of the fetus should be observed using tocometry, if available. Digital vaginal exams should be avoided, as manipulation of the placenta can cause significant hemorrhage.

Patients with significant or continuous hemorrhage will likely need a cesarean section to ultimately allow for source control of hemorrhage. In the case of an impending preterm cesarean section, the respiratory outcome of the fetus can be optimized by early administration of intramuscular betamethasone to the mother when gestational age is between 34 and 36 weeks. Mothers who are Rh negative should receive Rho(D) immune globin to prevent alloimmunization against any future pregnancies.

Consultation Considerations

An obstetrics consultation and evaluation are necessary for patients with placenta previa and active hemorrhage. If an obstetrics team is not available for in-person evaluation, the patient should be transferred to a facility that has both obstetric care and adequate blood bank services [1]. All patients with placenta previa who present with vaginal bleeding will require admission for further monitoring or treatment; treatment will depend on the severity of the patient's presentation and can vary from expectant management to emergent delivery with hysterectomy [13].

Emergency Department Course and Outcome

The patient's transabdominal ultrasound was concerning for placenta previa. She then received a transvaginal ultrasound that confirmed a complete anterior placenta previa with no evidence of vasa previa. A blood type and crossmatch for 2 units of packed red blood cells (PRBCs) was arranged. A bimanual exam was deferred due to risk of hemorrhage. Because this hospital does not have obstetric services and the patient was otherwise hemodynamically stable, she was ultimately accepted for transfer of care to the nearest hospital, where her personal obstetrician would be able to monitor her and intervene surgically as necessary. Unfortunately, because of a winter storm, flight transport was not available and ground ambulance transport which would typically take 45 minutes to an hour would now take 4–6 hours.

While waiting for the delayed ambulance, the patient remained in the emergency department receiving cardiorespiratory monitoring, serial hemoglobin and hematocrit evaluations, and continuous tocometry.

The patient continued to bleed, soaking approximately one pad per hour. Four hours after the initial levels, her hemoglobin was 10.5 g/dL, and her hematocrit was 30.2. Vital signs were unchanged after 1 L lactated Ringer's solution intravenous bolus, and the patient denied any new symptoms. Finally, the weather was improving, and one unit of PRBCs was hung prior to transport. The patient arrived at the accepting hospital without any complications.

At the receiving hospital, the bleeding eventually slowed, and the patient was admitted for bedrest, hemodynamic monitoring, and tocometry. She was given steroids for fetal lung maturation and eventually had a repeat cesarean section delivery at 36 weeks of gestation.

Key Points

- Ultrasound should always be performed prior to a speculum or digital exam when evaluating vaginal bleeding in the second or third trimester. Avoid digital exams if placenta previa is suspected, since manipulation of the placenta could cause massive hemorrhage.

- Transvaginal ultrasound is not contraindicated in placenta previa. Ultrasound findings may provide important prognostic information regarding placenta previa and the placenta accreta spectrum.
- Though obstetric services are necessary for management of placenta previa, the patient is best served at a facility where a cesarean section or even a hysterectomy (especially in the case of placenta accreta) can be performed.

References

1. Oyelese Y, Smulian JC. Placenta previa, placenta accreta, and vasa previa. Obstet Gynecol. 2006;107(4):927–41. https://doi.org/10.1097/01.AOG.0000207559.15715.98.
2. Faiz AS, Ananth CV. Etiology and risk factors for placenta previa: an overview and meta-analysis of observational studies. J Matern Fetal Neonatal Med. 2003;13(3):175–90. https://doi.org/10.1080/jmf.13.3.175.190.
3. Silver RM. Abnormal Placentation: Placenta Previa, Vasa Previa, and Placenta Accreta. Obstet Gynecol. 2015;126(3):654–68. https://doi.org/10.1097/AOG.0000000000001005.
4. Haeri S, Dildy GA 3rd. Maternal mortality from hemorrhage. Semin Perinatol. 2012;36(1):48–55. https://doi.org/10.1053/j.semperi.2011.09.010.
5. Ryu JM, Choi YS, Bae JY. Bleeding control using intrauterine continuous running suture during cesarean section in pregnant women with placenta previa. Arch Gynecol Obstet. 2019;299(1):135–9. https://doi.org/10.1007/s00404-018-4957-4.
6. Rao KP, Belogolovkin V, Yankowitz J, Spinnato JA 2nd. Abnormal placentation: evidence-based diagnosis and management of placenta previa, placenta accreta, and vasa previa. Obstet Gynecol Surv. 2012;67(8):503–19. https://doi.org/10.1097/OGX.0b013e3182685870.
7. Rosenberg T, Pariente G, Sergienko R, Wiznitzer A, Sheiner E. Critical analysis of risk factors and outcome of placenta previa. Arch Gynecol Obstet. 2011;284(1):47–51. https://doi.org/10.1007/s00404-010-1598-7.
8. DeLoughery E, Colwill AC, Edelman A, Samuelson BB. Red blood cell capacity of modern menstrual products: considerations for assessing heavy menstrual bleeding. BMJ Sex Reprod Health. 2023:bmjsrh-2023-201895. https://doi.org/10.1136/bmjsrh-2023-201895.
9. Timor-Tritsch IE, Monteagudo A, Cali G, et al. Cesarean scar pregnancy is a precursor of morbidly adherent placenta. Ultrasound Obstet Gynecol. 2014;44(3):346–53. https://doi.org/10.1002/uog.13426.
10. Feng Y, Li XY, Xiao J, et al. Relationship between placenta location and resolution of second trimester placenta previa. J Huazhong Univ Sci Technolog Med Sci. 2017;37(3):390–4. https://doi.org/10.1007/s11596-017-1745-5.
11. Jing L, Wei G, Mengfan S, Yanyan H. Effect of site of placentation on pregnancy outcomes in patients with placenta previa. PLoS One. 2018;13(7):e0200252. https://doi.org/10.1371/journal.pone.0200252.
12. Miller DA, Chollet JA, Goodwin TM. Clinical risk factors for placenta previa-placenta accreta. Am J Obstet Gynecol. 1997;177(1):210–4. https://doi.org/10.1016/s0002-9378(97)70463-0.
13. Findeklee S, Costa SD. Placenta accreta and total placenta previa in the 19th week of pregnancy. Geburtshilfe Frauenheilkd. 2015;75(8):839–43. https://doi.org/10.1055/s-0035-1557763.

Placental Abruption

It's Not a Big Deal, I Only Tripped

Marquita S. Norman, Jodi D. Jones, and Ava E. Pierce

Case

A 40-year-old G3P2 woman, 35 weeks pregnant, presents to the emergency department at 7:00 pm with her husband, who states that his wife tripped over a shoe and now has vaginal bleeding and severe abdominal pain. The patient reports that around 2:00 pm she was walking in her home, in her usual state of health, when she tripped over a shoe in the hallway, stumbled, and almost fell. Rather, she recalls that she stabilized herself against a wall, but did not fall or hit any other objects. She did not think she was injured, so she continued with her day. At 5:00 pm, she began to experience some contractions. Thinking they were Braxton Hicks contractions, she decided it was best to remain at home. At around 6:00 pm, she noticed the pain was persisting but now was accompanied by a small amount of vaginal bleeding.

- Past medical history: Hypertension
- Past surgical history: Two previous cesarean sections
- Medications: Hydralazine, prenatal vitamins
- Allergies: None
- Family history: Mother with hypertension; father with diabetes and coronary artery disease
- Social history: 10 pack-years of cigarette smoking history; quit smoking upon finding out that she was pregnant; no illicit drug use

M. S. Norman · J. D. Jones · A. E. Pierce (✉)
Department of Emergency Medicine, University of Texas Southwestern Medical Center, Dallas, TX, USA
e-mail: ava.pierce@utsouthwestern.edu

Physical Exam

- Vital signs
  - Heart rate: 90 beats/minute
  - Blood pressure: 100/70 mmHg
  - Respiratory rate: 18 breaths/minute
  - Temperature: 98 °F.
  - Oxygen saturation: 98% on room air
- General appearance: Well-nourished, gravid woman appearing in no acute distress
- HEENT
  - Head: Atraumatic, normocephalic
  - Eyes: Pupils equal, round, and reactive to light (4–2 mm); external ocular movements are normal; normal conjunctiva; no papilledema
  - Ears: No blood in external auditory canal, no hemotympanum
  - Nose: Within normal limits
  - Throat: No erythema or edema of the oropharynx
  - Neck: Trachea midline, no stridor, no jugular venous distention present
- Heart: Regular rate and rhythm, no murmur appreciated
- Lungs: Clear to auscultation bilaterally
- Abdominal/GI: Gravid with fundus above the umbilicus, mild tenderness in the suprapubic region
- Genitourinary: External exam shows blood on the outside of labia
- Rectal: Normal tone and brown stool
- Extremities: No tenderness, no edema
- Back: No midline tenderness, no costovertebral angle tenderness
- Neuro: CN II—XII grossly intact, 5/5 strength at bilateral upper and lower extremities, sensation intact, normal reflexes, no clonus
- Skin: Warm, dry, no rash
- Lymph: No palpable lymphadenopathy
- Psych: Normal affect and thought content

Pertinent Diagnostic Tests (Tables 6.1, 6.2, 6.3, 6.4 and 6.5)

Table 6.1 Complete blood count

Complete blood count	
White blood cells	16×10^9/L
Hemoglobin	11.2 g/dL
Hematocrit	33%
Platelets	250×10^9/L

Table 6.2 Comprehensive metabolic panel

Comprehensive metabolic panel	
Sodium	140 mEq/L
Potassium	4.0 mEq/L
Chloride	106 mEq/L
Bicarbonate	25 mEq/L
Glucose	98 mg/dL
Blood urea nitrogen (BUN)	8 mg/dL
Creatinine	0.8 mg/dL
Calcium	9.0 mg/dL
Total bilirubin	0.8 mg/dL
Alkaline phosphatase	80 units/L
Aspartate aminotransferase (AST)	36 units/L
Alanine aminotransferase (ALT)	38 units/L
Albumin	4 g/dL
Total protein	7.3 g/dL

Table 6.3 Venous blood gas and lactic acid

Venous blood gas and lactic acid	
pH	7.36
pCO2	42 mmHg
pO2	40 mmHg
HCO3	24 mEq/L
Lactic acid	2.6 mEq/L

Table 6.4 Coagulopathy panel

Coagulopathy panel	
International normalized ratio (INR)	1.0
Prothrombin time (PT)	12 seconds
Activated partial thromboplastin time (aPTT)	26 seconds

Table 6.5 Urinalysis

Urinalysis	
Color	Yellow
Appearance	Clear
Specific Gravity	6.0
pH	1.020
Glucose	Negative
Bilirubin	Negative
Ketones	0
Protein	1+
Leukocyte esterase	1+
Nitrites	Negative
White blood cells (WBCs)	2 WBCs/high-power field (HPF)
Red blood cells (RBCs)	2 RBCs/HPF
Squamous epithelial cells	0–3 cells/HPF

Learning Points

Background

Placental abruption (also called *abruptio placentae*) is a premature antenatal separation of the placenta (Fig. 6.1) from the endometrium that can result in compromised fetal perfusion. The most severe cases can result in maternal and/or fetal death. It is one of the more dangerous causes of vaginal bleeding during the second half of pregnancy and is due to traumatic injury or other weakening of the vessels which support the placenta. Maternal and fetal outcomes depend on the extent, location, and rate of separation. Risk factors for abruption include advanced maternal age, multiparity, recent traumatic injury, intrauterine infection, chronic hypertension, preeclampsia, in vitro fertilization (IVF), oligohydramnios, vascular disorders, premature birth, and consumption of tobacco, alcohol, or illicit drugs [1–3].

Placental abruption occurs secondary to maternal vessels tearing away from the placenta, causing bleeding to occur between the lining of the uterus and the maternal side of the placenta. The accumulation of blood in the new potential space causes the uterine wall to remain stable but the vascular structures of the connecting tissues to be injured. This can lead to hemodynamic instability, coagulation abnormalities, or acute fetal distress [1, 4].

Placental abruption is divided into classes based on clinical findings (Table 6.6). Class 1 is usually associated with a small degree of separation (partial or marginal),

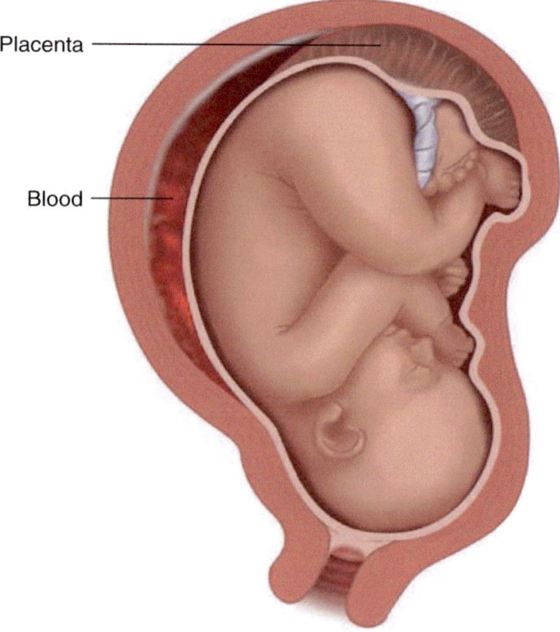

Fig. 6.1 Illustration of placental abruption, the placenta prematurely separating from the uterus

Table 6.6 Classification of placental abruption [4]

Placental abruption class	Clinical findings
Class 0: Asymptomatic	Discovery of a blood clot on the maternal side of a delivered placenta
Class 1: Mild	No vaginal bleeding or minimal vaginal bleeding
	Slight uterine tenderness
	Normal maternal blood pressure and heart rate
	No evidence of fetal distress
Class 2: Moderate	No vaginal bleeding to a moderate amount of vaginal bleeding
	Significant uterine tenderness with tetanic contractions
	Change in vital signs: maternal tachycardia, orthostatic changes in blood pressure
	Evidence of fetal distress
	Hypofibrinogenemia
Class 3: Severe	No vaginal bleeding to heavy vaginal bleeding
	Tetanic uterus/stiff uterine consistency on palpation
	Maternal shock
	Hypofibrinogenemia and coagulopathy
	Fetal death

and the patient is asymptomatic or has mild symptoms [4]. Class 2 or 3 are diagnosed with more severe symptoms (hemodynamic instability, fetal distress, or coagulopathy), due to complete or central separation [4].

Differential Diagnosis Subchorionic hemorrhage, placenta previa, uterine rupture, vasa previa, placenta accreta, placenta increta, placenta percreta.

History and Physical Exam

A diagnosis of placental abruption can only be made definitively by visualizing abnormal separation of the placenta from the uterus antepartum. Clinicians must rely on history and physical exam to consider placental abruption as a life-threatening cause of vaginal bleeding in the latter half of pregnancy. In particular, placental abruption is characterized by *painful* vaginal bleeding due to separation of the uterus from the placenta or from contractions of the uterus.

History should explore the patient's prenatal course to date and the general courses of any prior pregnancies. Placental abruption is a clinical diagnosis; therefore, a heightened clinical suspicion is indicated for pregnant patients presenting with low-energy mechanisms of injury. It is important to find out whether the patient has experienced any abdominal trauma, even if the patient considers that trauma to be minor in nature. A screen for intimate partner violence should be performed [5]. A social history will help risk-stratify the patient for placenta previa—specifically, identifying whether the patient has a history of smoking cigarettes or using cocaine. If the patient indeed has been having vaginal bleeding, an estimated blood loss and any associated pain should be noted. The patient should explain whether there have been contractions or if fetal movements have been noted.

The physical exam should always begin with an evaluation of the patient's vital signs. Hypotension or tachycardia could indicate shock due to placental abruption. The quantity of vaginal bleeding does not correlate with the severity of placental separation; the placenta can conceal a large abruption with no evidence of vaginal bleeding on pelvic exam [3]. The uterus should also be palpated for tenderness and for possible contractions. Specifically, when considering placental abruption, a digital cervical examination should not be performed before obtaining an ultrasound confirming the status of the placenta. A premature digital cervical exam could lead to catastrophic hemorrhage if the placenta is abnormally overlying the internal cervical os.

The fetal evaluation is the last portion of the physical exam that needs to be considered when evaluating for placental abruption. Increased suspicion for abruption arises with abnormal auscultation of fetal heart rate, i.e., <110 beats/minute or > 160 beats/minute, which can be obtained by Doppler or by bedside ultrasound. Continuous electronic fetal monitoring is preferred as soon as possible to evaluate for fetal distress by identifying bradycardia, late heart rate decelerations, or decreased of variability [5].

Laboratory Studies

There is no single laboratory test or testing pattern that is diagnostic for placental abruption. However, laboratory testing may be performed to help distinguish from other items in the differential diagnosis or to aid in management of the patient during the hospital stay [5].

A complete blood count, coagulation studies, and metabolic profile will help determine the patient's baseline status. A blood type and Rh screen should be performed in case a blood transfusion is necessary and to determine whether a patient should receive Rh factor given the possible exchange of fetal and maternal blood fluids. A urinalysis may reveal proteinuria, which is not uncommon in cases of placental abruption [1, 4].

A Kleihauer–Betke test can be performed to evaluate for fetal blood in maternal circulation. This can suggest placental abruption but is not diagnostic. For Rh-negative patients, a positive test could suggest isoimmunization and confirm a need for Rh(D) immunoglobulin administration [5].

Imaging Findings

Although ultrasonography is recommended for all patients suspected of placental abruption to evaluate for a viable intrauterine pregnancy and to evaluate the surrounding maternal-fetal structures, placental abruption is primarily a clinical diagnosis. The bleeding associated with an acute placental abruption may be small or minimally echoic compared to the surrounding placental tissue, making an abruption difficult to visualize [1]. Pressure of the transducer may cause accumulated clotted blood to tremble, which is known as the "Jell-O sign." It typically takes about one week for a hematoma to become hypoechoic and at about two weeks, the hematoma appears sonolucent [2, 6], making it easier to distinguish from the placenta. As the ultrasound findings of hematoma and hemorrhage for placental abruption are variable, depending on the size, age, and location of the abruption, ultrasonography is specific when the hemorrhage is visualized but not reliable or sensitive when diagnosing placental abruption. An ultrasound interpreted as "normal" does not rule out placental abruption.

Management

If strongly considered as the likely diagnosis, placental abruption typically requires immediate intervention for best outcomes for both the patient and the fetus. Intravenous access should be initiated and if the patient is experiencing signs of hemorrhage or hemorrhagic shock, the patient should receive intravenous fluids and/or blood products to prevent decompensation. Supplemental oxygen should also be considered. If signs of distress are identified by continuous maternal or fetal monitoring, care will need to be escalated [4].

If the patient's presentation suggests a mild placental abruption (e.g., class 0 or 1) and the patient is clinically stable, the patient may be observed in the hospital for any clinical changes or until the fetus is mature enough for safe delivery [4]. Administration of betamethasone 12 mg or dexamethasone 6 mg intramuscularly to the patient should be considered early to promote lung development in the fetus, with dexamethasone having a faster onset but a shorter half-life [7].

If the patient seems to be experiencing a more severe placental abruption (e.g., class 2 or 3), and the fetus is viable, emergency delivery should occur either vaginally by induction of labor or by cesarean section. A vaginal delivery may be safer for the mother by lessening the chances of critical hemorrhage, but a cesarean section birth may decrease the changes of circulatory compromise to the fetus. If, at any time, the fetus is demonstrating signs of distress, an emergency cesarean section is the preferred mechanism of delivery [4]. Rho(D) immune globulin should be strongly considered (300 mcg IM) for Rh-negative patients to prevent isoimmunization affecting future pregnancies [4, 5].

Consultation Considerations

An emergent obstetrics consultation is indicated when a placental abruption is suspected. Any inpatient observation will typically be carried out by an obstetrics service. If there are signs of active hemorrhage or fetal distress, an obstetrician should facilitate delivery of the fetus. Hematology consultation should be considered for any coagulopathies which may be identified, potentially complicating the course of placental abruption [4, 5].

Emergency Department Course and Outcome

Upon discovery of vaginal bleeding in this high-risk third trimester pregnancy, the obstetrics team was consulted emergently.

A bedside point of care ultrasound by the emergency physician revealed an intrauterine pregnancy of approximately 35 weeks' age, with a heart rate of 155 beats/minute with minimal hyperechoic fluid between the placenta and myometrium.

The obstetrics team ordered a STAT portable ultrasound to be performed by the radiology department. The radiologist called with concern that, though the placenta seemed intact, there was a non-vascular heterogeneous area measuring 4 cm between the placenta and myometrium, suspicious for placental abruption.

The patient was admitted to the labor and delivery unit for continuous fetal monitoring. The initial cardiotocography revealed a fetal heart rate of 150–160 beats/minute. One hour later, the patient complained of worsening abdominal pain. A repeat physical examination revealed increased uterine tenderness. The patient's blood pressure decreased to 90/60 mmHg, and heart rate increased to 120 beats/minute. The fetal heart rate increased to 180 beats/minute, and the team appreciated late decelerations on continuous monitoring.

The patient was taken to the operating room for emergent cesarean section under general anesthesia. During delivery, the patient received a transfusion of 2 units packed red blood cells, which normalized the patient's vital signs. The baby was delivered, requiring only simple stimulation, and was admitted to the neonatal intensive care unit. The mother was admitted to the intensive care unit overnight for monitoring and eventually transferred to the general obstetric floor. Both mother and baby were discharged from the hospital in stable condition on hospital day 4.

Key Points

- Clinical suspicion for placental abruption should be high in any case of trauma, even if the injury was a relatively low-energy mechanism.
- Placental abruption is a clinical diagnosis; ultrasound may be useful, but sensitivity is poor.
- The amount of vaginal bleeding does not correlate well with the severity of placental separation.
- Early continuous fetal monitoring is important to determine fetal distress that might require emergency cesarean section.

References

1. Alouini S, Valery A, Lemaire B, Evrard ML, Belin O. Diagnosis and management of pregnant women with placental abruption and neonatal outcomes. Cureus. 2022;14(1):e21120. https://doi.org/10.7759/cureus.21120

2. Shih P, Tsai TY, Gozari G. Pregnant woman with vaginal bleeding. Ann Emerg Med. 2021;77(1):125–37. https://doi.org/10.1016/j.annemergmed.2020.07.019.
3. Young JS, White LM. Vaginal bleeding in late pregnancy. Emerg Med Clin North Am. 2019;37(2):251–64. https://doi.org/10.1016/j.emc.2019.01.006.
4. Schmidt P, Skelly CL, Raines DA. Placental abruption. In: StatPearls. Treasure Island: StatPearls Publishing; 1 Apr 2022. Available from: https://www.ncbi.nlm.nih.gov/books/NBK482335/
5. Huls CK, Detlefs C. Trauma in pregnancy. Semin Perinatol. 2018;42(1):13–20. https://doi.org/10.1053/j.semperi.2017.11.004.
6. Suzuki R, Furuya N, Hasegawa J, Homma C, Iwahata Y, Suzuki N. Ultrasonographic findings of placental abruption observed on superb microvascular imaging. Taiwan J Obstet Gynecol. 2022;61(4):713–6. https://doi.org/10.1016/j.tjog.2021.08.007.
7. Emeruwa UN, Krenitsky NM, Sheen JJ. Advances in management for preterm fetuses at risk of delivery. Clin Perinatol. 2020;47(4):685–703. https://doi.org/10.1016/j.clp.2020.08.006.

Asymptomatic Hypertension in Pregnancy

A New High

Felisha Perry-Smith and Adeola A. Kosoko

Case

A 36-year-old woman, G2P1 at 21 weeks' gestation, presents to the emergency department (ED) with a complaint of "hypertension." She was getting a routine dental cleaning this morning, and the dentist recommended that she should be evaluated by a physician as soon as possible to follow up on the routine blood pressure measurement obtained during the visit, which was "too high," at 159/73 mmHg. The patient remarks that she has had a normal pregnancy to date and that she is afraid of what this diagnosis could mean for her and her baby. She denies any other complaints.

- Past medical history: Regular prenatal care, normal prenatal course to date, no history of miscarriages, abortions, or premature births; obesity (body mass index of 32).
- Past surgical history: None.
- Medications: Prenatal vitamins.
- Allergies: No known drug allergies.
- Family history: Mother with insulin-dependent diabetes mellitus and hypertension, father with hypertension.
- Social history: Non-smoker, no alcohol, no illicit drug use.

Supplementary Information The online version contains supplementary material available at https://doi.org/10.1007/978-3-031-70118-4_7.

F. Perry-Smith · A. A. Kosoko (✉)
Department of Emergency Medicine, McGovern School of Medicine, University of Texas Health Sciences Center at Houston, Houston, TX, USA
e-mail: Adeola.A.Kosoko@uth.tmc.edu

Physical Exam

- Vital signs
  - Heart rate: 92 beats/minute
  - Blood pressure: 164/85 mmHg
  - Respiratory rate: 16 breaths/minute
  - Temperature 98.8 °F
  - Oxygen saturation: 99% on room air

- General appearance: No acute distress; appears stated age, well-nourished
- HEENT
  - Head/neck: Normocephalic, atraumatic, supple
  - Eyes: Normal extraocular movements, pupils equal and reactive, conjunctiva normal
  - Ears/Nose/throat: Mucus membranes moist, oropharynx clear

- Heart: Regular rate, rhythm, no peripheral edema
- Lungs: Normal respiratory effort, speaks in full sentences, no accessory muscle use, clear to auscultation without rhonchi, wheezes, or rales
- Abdominal/GI: Soft, nontender, nondistended, no pulsatile masses, no fluid wave, uterine fundus palpable at the umbilicus
- Extremities: Normal range of motion, no edema
- Neuro: Speech is clear and appropriate, normal level of consciousness, gait and coordination are normal, 5/5 strength in all extremities
- Skin: Warm; normal color; no rashes, dermatoses, petechiae, or lesions
- Psych: Normal mood and effect, judgment/competence is appropriate

Pertinent Diagnostic Tests (Figs. 7.1 and 7.2a,b,c, Tables 7.1, 7.2 and 7.3)

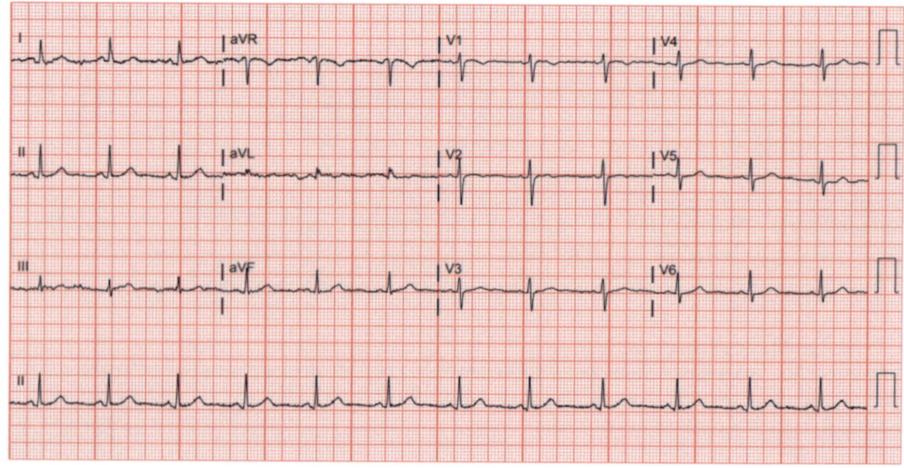

Fig. 7.1 Electrocardiogram (ECG): Normal sinus rhythm . (F. Perry-Smith's own image)

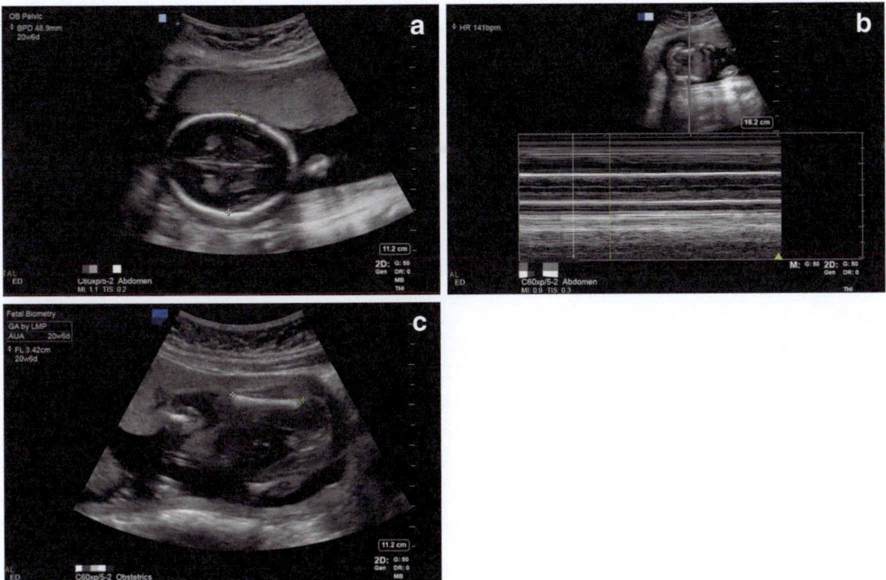

Fig. 7.2 Point-of-care transabdominal ultrasound (**a**) Biparietal diameter, (**b**) Fetal heart rate, (**c**) Femur length: Intrauterine pregnancy at 20 weeks and 6 days and fetal heart rate of 141 beats per minute. (Images courtesy of C. Bakunas and R. Bower)

Table 7.1 Complete blood count

Complete blood count	
White blood cells	4.8×0^9/L
Hemoglobin	12.9 g/dL
Hematocrit	39%
Platelets	223×10^9/L

Table 7.2 Comprehensive metabolic panel

Comprehensive metabolic panel	
Sodium	138 mEq/L
Potassium	4.1 mEq/L
Chloride	102 mEq/L
Bicarbonate	24 mEq/L
Glucose	88 mg/dL
Blood urea nitrogen (BUN)	13 mg/dL
Creatinine	0.9 mg/dL
Calcium	8.9 mg/dL
Total bilirubin	0.95 mg/dL
Alkaline phosphatase	95 units/L
Aspartate aminotransferase (AST)	19 units/L
Alanine aminotransferase (ALT)	15 units/L
Albumin	3.5 g/dL
Total protein	7.0 g/dL

Table 7.3 Urinalysis

Urinalysis	
Color	Yellow
Appearance	Clear
Specific Gravity	1.012
pH	5.2
Glucose	15 mg/dL
Bilirubin	Negative
Ketones	None
Protein	15 mg/dL
Leukocyte esterase	Negative
Nitrites	Negative
White blood cells (WBCs)	2 WBCs/High-Power Field (HPF)
Red blood cells (RBCs)	0 RBCs/HPF
Squamous epithelial cells	0–5 cells/HPF
Bacteria	None
Yeast	None

Table 7.4 Classifications of severity of hypertension in pregnancy

	Systolic blood pressure	And	Diastolic blood pressure
Mild	140–149 mmHg	And	90–99 mmHg
Moderate	150–159 mmHg	And	100–109 mmHg
Severe	$\geq$ 160 mmHg	And	$\geq$ 110 mmHg

Learning Points

Background

Hypertension affects 6–10% of pregnant persons in the United States. Hypertension in pregnancy is defined as a systolic blood pressure (BP) $\geq$ 140 mmHg and diastolic $\geq$90 mmHg, for two separate measurements taken at least four hours apart. There are three classifications of hypertension in pregnancy (Table 7.4).

Hypertension during pregnancy exists as a continuum, from pre-existing hypertension (or chronic hypertension) to preeclampsia. Pre-existing hypertension (i.e., hypertension in a non-pregnant patient) is defined as BP $\geq$ 140/90 on two separate occasions *before* 20 weeks gestational age (WGA) or lasting greater than 12 weeks postpartum. Typically, a pregnant state does not worsen a pre-existing condition of hypertension. Gestational hypertension is defined as blood pressure greater than or equal to 140 mmHg systolic or 90 mmHg diastolic on two separate occasions at least 4 hours apart after 20 weeks of pregnancy when previous blood pressure measurements were normal. There should not be associated signs or symptoms of eclampsia or preeclampsia and after delivery of the baby, the blood pressure should return to normal [1].

Similarly, if ever the patient's systolic blood pressure is greater than 160 mmHg or diastolic blood pressure is greater than 110 mmHg in a single measurement (i.e., severe hypertension), gestational hypertension is confirmed if the blood pressure is reproducible even after a short interval [2]. A patient is reclassified to chronic hypertension if elevated blood pressures persist longer than 12 weeks postpartum. Preeclampsia and eclampsia are considered hypertensive emergencies of pregnancy. Preeclampsia is defined as BP $\geq$ 140/90 on two separate occasions at least 4 hours apart *after* 20 WGA. It is often associated with signs of end organ damage, visual changes, or right upper quadrant/epigastric pain. Hypertension related to preeclampsia is typically rather abrupt in onset.

Blood pressure measurements must be interpreted in the context of each trimester of pregnancy. In the first trimester, blood pressure tends to be lower, typically reaching the lowest point mid-pregnancy, around 20 weeks, and then rising again until delivery [3]. Blood pressure levels typically return to preconception levels by the third trimester.

Hypertension in pregnancy is multifactorial, and the pathogenic mechanism is not yet fully understood.

Differential Diagnosis pre-existing (chronic) hypertension, gestational hypertension, preeclampsia, HELLP (hemolysis, elevated liver enzymes, and low platelets) syndrome, unclassifiable hypertension.

History and Physical Exam

The asymptomatic patient will usually present to the ED at the behest of a medical professional who obtained an abnormally high blood pressure measurement (e.g., a nurse, dentist, midwife, or physician) or because the patient or some other well-meaning person measured the blood pressure and found it abnormal. An asymptomatic patient, by definition, should deny any associated symptoms (e.g., headache, blurred vision, or right upper quadrant or epigastric pain) when presenting with the chief complaint of elevated blood pressure. She should also have a confirmed pregnant state. Most importantly, the patient should share any blood pressure measurements and timing of the measurements when providing a pertinent history for hypertension.

Invasive blood pressure measurement (i.e., arterial catheter measurement) is the gold standard of measuring blood pressure. However, electronic blood pressure measurements are typically used as a general screen of blood pressure. The accuracy of electronic blood pressure measurements depends on the proper calibration of the machine. The mainstay of generally accurate measurements of blood pressure is the use of a manual sphygmomanometer and stethoscope. Proper blood pressure measurement technique ideally involves having the patient in seated position, uncrossed legs, back supported or in left lateral decubitus, and utilizing a properly sized cuff. The patient should also have rested for 10 minutes and abstained from tobacco or caffeine use for 30 minutes prior to measurement. Ideally, blood pressure should be taken in both arms and both documented.

Asymptomatic hypertension in the pregnant patient should also document lack of concerning physical exam signs. The presence of increasing peripheral edema could be concerning for preeclampsia. Rales, dyspnea, or jugular venous distention would suggest pulmonary edema and could be highly concerning for heart failure. A neurologic exam should be normal. The abdomen should not be tender. Specifically, right upper quadrant pain could suggest HELLP syndrome.

It is important to differentiate between a pregnant woman presenting to the ED with asymptomatic hypertension and other populations that may present with asymptomatic hypertension. The pregnant population is at significantly increased risk for poor outcomes for mother and child if the hypertension is not identified and addressed. Therefore, unlike other asymptomatic patients presenting to the ED with concern for hypertension, the asymptomatic pregnant patient routinely requires a more extensive evaluation.

Laboratory Studies

Laboratory studies for the hypertensive pregnant patient should be routinely performed in the ED to identify any non-pregnancy causes of hypertension and to identify any complications of hypertension which could potentially adversely affect the mother or the fetus. Specifically, risk stratification by laboratory testing should be performed for patients >20 WGA to evaluate for preeclampsia or HELLP syndrome.

A random clean-catch urine sample should be sent for urinalysis. A urine protein of >30 mg/dL (commonly 1+ on a urine dipstick) is sufficient in the ED to evaluate for proteinuria, though the gold standard is a 24-hour urine collection. A complete blood count would particularly evaluate for thrombocytopenia (platelets $<100 \times 10^9/L$). A complete metabolic panel will evaluate for renal function and hepatic function. Serum creatinine >1.1 mg/dL or a value double the baseline creatinine (in absence of other renal disease) suggests renal injury. Transaminase levels greater than twice the normal limits suggest hepatic injury.

Imaging Findings

There are no imaging studies indicated or recommended for diagnosis of asymptomatic hypertension in pregnancy. Pelvic ultrasound may be obtained to assess the wellbeing of the fetus (Fig. 7.3).

It is not recommended to obtain routine ECGs for asymptomatic patients with hypertension. Typical physiologic adaptations during pregnancy include an increased heart rate, cardiac output, and intravascular volume. In return, expected changes noted on an ECG can include sinus tachycardia, left axis deviation, ectopic beats, flattened or inverted T-waves, and/or a Q-wave in lead III [4].

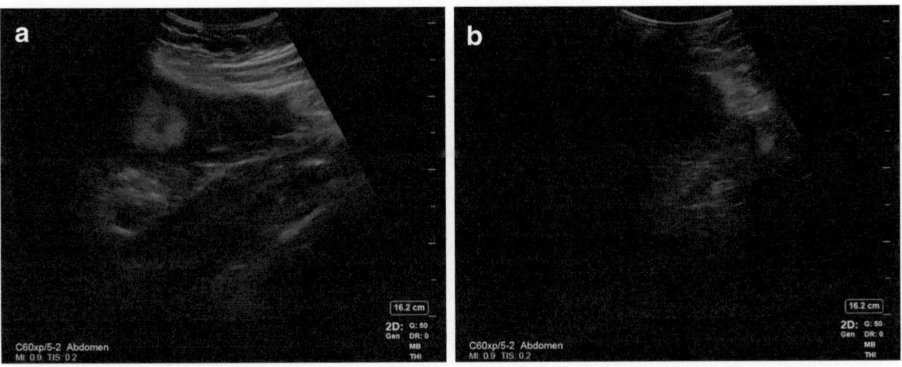

Fig. 7.3 Point-of-Care transabdominal ultrasound (**a**) Long view, (**b**) Short view: Normal intra-uterine pregnancy at 20 weeks and 6 days gestational age. (Images courtesy of C. Bakunas, MD and R. Bower, MD)

Management

Treatment of severe hypertension in pregnancy (>160/110 mmHg)—whether gestational hypertension or chronic hypertension—is always indicated, most readily using pharmaceutical agents. Chronic hypertension diagnosed and treated prior to pregnancy should continue to be treated through pregnancy, making sure that the agents prescribed are safe for use during pregnancy [5, 6].

Therapeutic guidelines vary among different obstetric and medical societies due to lack of evidence supporting a blood pressure goal [6, 7]. Professional society guidelines range between blood pressure goals of 120–160 mmHg and 130–155 mmHg systolic and 80–105 mmHg diastolic in healthy populations without other comorbidities. In all patients with comorbidities, such as renal disease, proteinuria, left ventricular hypertrophy, hypertensive retinopathy, microvascular disease, stroke, and age greater than 40, initiate antihypertensive therapy for diastolic BP $\geq$ 90 mmHg.

The United States Food and Drug Administration (FDA) is tasked with classifying drugs according to their risk when taken during pregnancy. In 2015, the FDA implemented a more specific system to improve decision-making for drug prescriptions, called the Pregnancy and Lactation Labeling Rule (PLLR). The PLLR is available with all prescription drug labels, with more specific information on risk relating to pregnancy, lactation, and for males and females who have the potential to reproduce [8]. However, most physicians rely on the bygone standard pregnancy-risk category system utilized by the FDA in determining drug choices (Table 7.5) [8]. No antihypertensive medications carry a category A classification due to the lack of randomized controlled trials to evaluate these medications in pregnant human subjects. Therefore, most prescribed medications in pregnancy carry class B and class C classifications [9].

Table 7.5 FDA pregnancy-risk categories [8]

Category A	No risk in human studies (studies in pregnant women have not demonstrated a risk to the fetus during the first trimester).
Category B	No risk in animal studies (there are no adequate studies in humans, but animal studies did not demonstrate a risk to the fetus).
Category C	Risk cannot be ruled out. There are no satisfactory studies in pregnant women, but animal studies demonstrated a risk to the fetus; potential benefits of the drug may outweigh the risks.
Category D	Evidence of risk (studies in pregnant women have demonstrated a risk to the fetus; potential benefits of the drug may outweigh the risks).
Category X	Contraindicated (studies in pregnant women have demonstrated a risk to the fetus, and/or human or animal studies have shown fetal abnormalities; risks of the drug outweigh the potential benefits).

Initiation of monotherapy with an accepted first-line oral antihypertensive agent is the recommended treatment. First-line antihypertensives in pregnancy include labetalol, nifedipine, and methyldopa [6]. Methyldopa (class B), a central alpha-adrenergic agonist, has a long history of use in pregnancy due to proven long-term safety and efficacy. However, present-day, methyldopa is less frequently used compared to calcium channel blockers (CCB) or beta blockers which are also currently first line, more efficient, and require less frequent dosing [10, 11]. Some patients may not tolerate methyldopa due to the side effects of somnolence and postural hypotension. The peak effect of methyldopa is seen 2–3 hours after administration and maximum effect after 4–6 hours. The total daily dose is 500 mg divided into 2–3 daily oral doses [5, 9].

Labetalol (class C), an $alpha_1$-adrenergic blocker and a nonselective beta-adrenergic blocker (beta:alpha blockade ratio of 7:1), has comparable efficacy to methyldopa and is recommended as a first-line agent against hypertension in pregnancy [5, 6, 9]. The American College of Obstetricians and Gynecologists (ACOG) recommends against using labetalol in women with asthma, myocardial disease, decreased cardiac function, heart block, or bradycardia due to the possible adverse beta-blockade effects [9]. The typical starting dose is 100 mg two times per day, which can be increased weekly outpatient to a maximum 2400 mg daily [5, 9].

Nifedipine (class C), a CCB, was formerly considered second line or alternative first line, but presently it is a preferred first-line agent [5, 6, 9]. However, the data supporting nifedipine is not as abundant as that for methyldopa or labetalol. Prescribing a long-acting medication may improve patient adherence, and nifedipine is dosed once daily. The typical starting dose is 30 mg daily and can be increased to 60–90 mg daily outpatient [5, 9, 12]. The sublingual route of nifedipine can lead to less predictable blood levels and is generally not the preferred dosing route.

More recent guidelines have acknowledged that in women with salt-sensitive chronic hypertension or chronic kidney disease and reduced glomerular filtration rate, diuretics may be used safely during pregnancy to treat hypertension, although perhaps at lower doses [6]. Furosemide (class C) and hydrochlorothiazide (class C) are considered second-line antihypertensives during pregnancy [5]. The preferred diuretic, according to ACOG, is hydrochlorothiazide with a recommended starting dose of 12.5–25 mg per day [5]. Reduction in intravascular volume leading to decreased uteroplacental flow is a theoretical side effect of diuretic use in pregnancy; however, this has not been proven to be clinically significant [10]. In the setting of persistent hypertension or chronic hypertension, patients may continue their home thiazide diuretics. Spironolactone, which is a diuretic and an aldosterone antagonist, should not be used in pregnancy, especially the first trimester, due to possible fetal anti-androgen effects, also known as feminization effects [7, 12].

Hydralazine is a vasodilator that can be considered for use as a monotherapy; however, there is the side effect of reflexive tachycardia. The shorter half-life of hydralazine also requires more frequent dosing, which may challenge patient adherence. Dosing for hydralazine begins at 10 mg three times per day to four times per day with a maximum 300 mg per day [12].

Nicardipine and clonidine are less extensively researched agents in pregnancy and may be considered for resistant hypertension [5, 6, 12].

Angiotensin-converting enzyme inhibitors (ACE inhibitors) and angiotensin II antagonists are contraindicated in pregnancy due to their proven teratogenic effects (class C in first trimester and class D in third trimester) (Table 7.6) [5, 9, 11, 12].

When a patient is experiencing severe hypertension, labetalol, nifedipine, or hydralazine is typically used to lower blood pressure with repeated doses as necessary to achieve a blood pressure goal.

Definitive management for gestational hypertension is delivery of the fetus [5, 9]. Until then, close, and frequent monitoring of blood pressure and

Table 7.6 Preferred antihypertensive agents during pregnancy

	Drug class	Drug name	Dosing	Pregnancy-risk category
First line	Beta agonists	Labetalol	100 mg twice daily (daily maximum 2400 mg)	C
	Calcium channel blockers	Nifedipine	30–60 mg daily (daily maximum 120 mg)	C
	Vasodilators/ nitrates	Hydralazine	10 mg 3 times daily (daily maximum 120 mg)	C
	Alpha agonists	Methyldopa	250 mg 2–3 times daily (daily maximum 3000 mg)	B
Second line	Alpha agonists	Clonidine	0.1 mg 1–2 times daily (daily maximum 0.3 mg)	C
	Thiazide diuretics	Hydrochlorothiazide	25–50 mg daily (daily maximum 50 mg)	C

Contraindicated
Angiotensin-converting enzyme (ACE) Inhibitors
Angiotensin II receptor blockers (ARBs)
Direct renin inhibitors
Nitroprusside
Spironolactone

laboratory testing will be required for the patient. This is typically managed in the outpatient setting.

Ideally, prevention of hypertension would be the goal for the pregnant patient. Studies have shown that treatment of non-severe hypertension in pregnancy is of benefit to the mother and is without associated perinatal risk [11]. Treating hypertension with antihypertensive agents during pregnancy may also prevent chronic hypertension progressing to severe hypertension. However, fetal complications such as intrauterine growth restriction, placental abruption, and preeclampsia are not necessarily reduced [6, 9]. Negative side effects (of appropriate antihypertensive therapy) on the fetus have not been consistently supported [6, 13].

Non-pharmacological treatment, such as lifestyle modification, is suggested as treatment in women with mild to moderate hypertension during pregnancy. However, there has been no evidence of prevention of hypertension with initiation of an exercise regimen during pregnancy. Obesity on its own is a risk factor for gestational hypertension. Therefore, it is important for pregnant women to adhere to the established recommendations for expectant gestational weight gain. Per the Institute of Medicine, body mass index (BMI) recommendations for weight gain during pregnancy based on pre-pregnancy weight currently dictate that patient with BMI 18.5–24.9 gain 25–35 pounds, while overweight patients (BMI 25–29.9) gain 15–25 pounds, and obese patients (BMI >30) gain 11–20 pounds [14]. However, BMI as a general marker of healthy weight is only a guideline presently. BMI as a ubiquitous standard has undergone significant scrutiny regarding its accuracy for all types of bodies because it does not sufficiently consider individual fat levels, body frame, muscle mass, or weight distribution.

Consultation Considerations

An obstetric or gynecologic (Ob/Gyn) consultation should be made for any patient who may require admission for acute, severe blood pressure, or patients who develop symptoms or who meet criteria for preeclampsia or end organ damage. Otherwise, if discharging a patient with hypertension, Ob/Gyn follow-up is important to promote optimal outcomes for both the mother and baby by monitoring and adjusting an antihypertensive regimen. Not all family medicine physicians or internal medicine physicians may be comfortable with the management of hypertension in pregnancy. Frequency of evaluation depends on the severity of the hypertensive disorder identified [5].

Consider outpatient cardiology follow-up for patients with more complex cardiovascular disease and hypertension in pregnancy.

ACOG recommends monitoring blood pressure in the hospital setting for 4–8 hours to distinguish acute severe elevations from transient elevations [5]. For discharged patients, ACOG recommends home blood pressure monitoring [5].

Emergency Department Course and Outcome

The patient good-naturedly waited for the results of her laboratory studies. Once completed, the emergency physician reviewed the laboratory tests with her. Nursing rechecked her blood pressure at 4 hours which was 153/70 mmHg. The physician explained concern for asymptomatic gestational hypertension. The patient did not have severe hypertension or signs of preeclampsia, HELLP, or end organ damage.

The emergency physician discussed the case with the patient's outpatient obstetrician by telephone. The obstetrician recommended the patient would be a good candidate for taking a low dose of labetalol, 100 mg orally, twice daily. The patient understood the diagnosis and felt comfortable with her plan of care. She would keep a blood pressure journal at home and visit the clinic for a reassessment in 7–10 days.

Key Points

- Though asymptomatic hypertension does not require an emergency department workup for the general population, several screening measures are indicated for the gravid patient.
- Nifedipine, labetalol, and methyldopa are first-line agents for management of hypertension in pregnancy.
- Angiotensin-converting enzyme (ACE) inhibitors, angiotensin receptor blockers (ARBs), and spironolactone are contraindicated for blood pressure management in the gravid patient.

References

1. Cunningham GF, editor. Williams obstetrics. 24th ed. New York: McGraw-Hill Professional; 2014.
2. Wiles K, Damodaram M, Frise C. Severe hypertension in pregnancy. Clin Med (Lond). 2021;21(5):e451–6. https://doi.org/10.7861/clinmed.2021-0508.
3. Ochsenbein-Kölble N, Roos M, Gasser T, Huch R, Huch A, Zimmermann R. Cross sectional study of automated blood pressure measurements throughout pregnancy. BJOG. 2004;111(4):319–25. https://doi.org/10.1111/j.1471-0528.2004.00099.x.
4. Angeli F, Angeli E, Verdecchia P. Electrocardiographic changes in hypertensive disorders of pregnancy. Hypertens Res. 2014;37(11):973–5. https://doi.org/10.1038/hr.2014.128.
5. American College of Obstetricians and Gynecologists' Committee on Practice Bulletins—Obstetrics. ACOG practice bulletin no. 203: chronic hypertension in pregnancy. Obstet Gynecol. 2019;133(1):e26–50. https://doi.org/10.1097/aog.0000000000003020.
6. Garovic VD, Dechend R, Easterling T, Karumanchi SA, McMurtry Baird S, Magee LA, et al. Hypertension in pregnancy: diagnosis, blood pressure goals, and pharmacotherapy: a scientific statement from the American Heart Association. Hypertension. 2022;79(2):e21–41. https://doi.org/10.1161/hyp.0000000000000208.
7. Kintiraki E, Papakatsika S, Kotronis G, Goulis DG, Kotsis V. Pregnancy-induced hypertension. Hormones (Athens). 2015;14(2):211–23. https://doi.org/10.14310/horm.2002.1582.

8. Leek JC, Arif H. Pregnancy medications. [Updated 24 Jul 2023]. In: StatPearls [internet]. Treasure Island: StatPearls Publishing; 2023. Available from: https://www.ncbi.nlm.nih.gov/books/NBK507858/

9. Rosner JY, Mehta-Lee SS. Hypertension in pregnancy. In: DeCherney AH, editor. Current diagnosis & treatment: obstetrics & gynecology. 12th ed. New York: McGraw Hill Education; 2019.

10. Kattah AG, Garovic VD. The management of hypertension in pregnancy. Adv Chronic Kidney Dis. 2013;20(3):229–39. https://doi.org/10.1053/j.ackd.2013.01.014.

11. Lai C, Coulter SA, Woodruff A. Hypertension and pregnancy. Tex Heart Inst J. 2017;44(5):350–1. https://doi.org/10.14503/thij-17-6359.

12. Kaye AB, Bhakta A, Moseley AD, Rao AK, Arif S, Lichtenstein SJ, et al. Review of cardiovascular drugs in pregnancy. J Womens Health (Larchmt). 2019;28(5):686–97. https://doi.org/10.1089/jwh.2018.7145.

13. Halpern DG, Weinberg CR, Pinnelas R, Mehta-Lee S, Economy KE, Valente AM. Use of medication for cardiovascular disease during pregnancy: JACC state-of-the-art review. J Am Coll Cardiol. 2019;73(4):457–76. https://doi.org/10.1016/j.jacc.2018.10.075.

14. Institute of Medicine (US) and National Research Council (US) committee to reexamine IOM pregnancy weight guidelines. In: Rasmussen KM, Yaktine AL, editors. Weight gain during pregnancy: reexamining the guidelines. Washington, DC: National Academies Press (US); 2009.

Preeclampsia and Eclampsia

A Shake and a Stir

Valerie A. Pierre

Case

A 39-year-old woman, G1P1 and 2 weeks postpartum, is brought in by emergency medical services (EMS) for a gradually worsening headache and blurry vision for one day. Her husband states that she took acetaminophen with little improvement of her symptoms. He encouraged her to come to the emergency department (ED) after her condition seemed to worsen with a transient episode of confusion and shortness of breath while walking to the bathroom. He reports that she recently had an uncomplicated pregnancy with a normal spontaneous vaginal delivery of a healthy baby boy and was in her normal state of health until today.

- Past medical history: Type 1 diabetes mellitus
- Past surgical history: None
- Medications: Sliding scale insulin
- Allergies: No known drug allergies
- Family history: Hypertension in mother
- Social history: Non-smoker. No alcohol use. No illicit drug use.

Physical Exam

- Vital signs
  - Heart rate: 112 beats/minute
  - Blood pressure: 226/107 mmHg
  - Respiratory rate: 20 breaths/minute

V. A. Pierre (✉)
Department of Emergency Medicine, University of Maryland School of Medicine, Baltimore, MD, USA
e-mail: valerie.pierre@som.umaryland.edu

A. A. Kosoko (ed.), *Emergency Medicine Case-Based Guide*,
https://doi.org/10.1007/978-3-031-70118-4_8

- – Temperature: 98.6 °F
- – Oxygen saturation: 93% on room air
- General appearance: Appears as stated age, lying supine on the stretcher, appears uncomfortable
- HEENT
  - – Head: Atraumatic, normocephalic
  - – Eyes: Pupils equal, round, reactive to light; blurred disc margins on fundoscopy
  - – Ears: Within normal limits
  - – Nose: Within normal limits
  - – Throat: No erythema or edema of the oropharynx
  - – Neck: Trachea midline, no stridor, jugular venous distention present
- Heart: Tachycardia, regular rhythm, equal pulses
- Lungs: Slightly tachypneic, absence of retractions, absence of rales
- Abdominal: Soft, boggy, nontender, bowel sounds present, consistent with post-partum status
- Genitourinary: Normal external genitalia, no vaginal bleeding, internal exam deferred
- Extremities: 1+ pitting edema in bilateral lower extremities, no tenderness, no deformity, tolerates full range of motion, negative Homan's sign bilaterally
- Back: Normal
- Neuro: Awake, alert and oriented x 4, follows simple commands
- Skin: Normal
- Psych: Normal

Pertinent Diagnostic Tests (Figs. 8.1 and 8.2, Tables 8.1, 8.2, 8.3, 8.4, 8.5, 8.6 and 8.7)

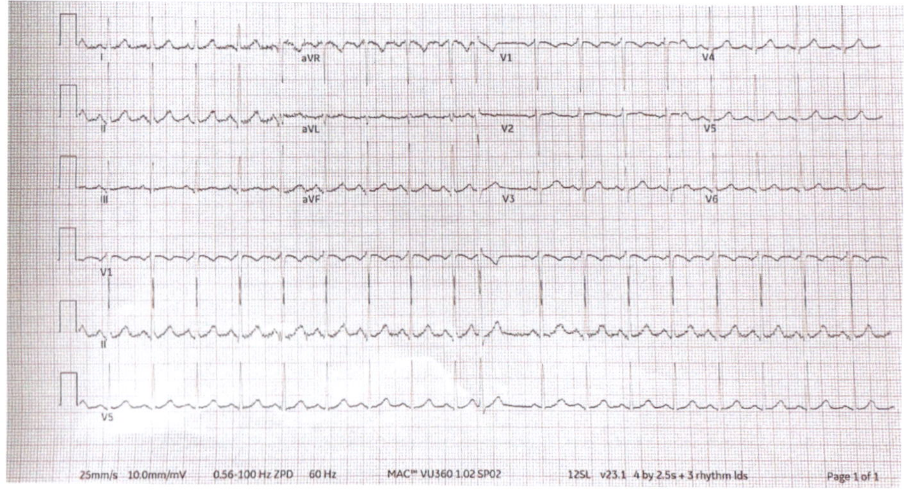

Fig. 8.1 Electrocardiogram (ECG): Sinus tachycardia (Author's own image)

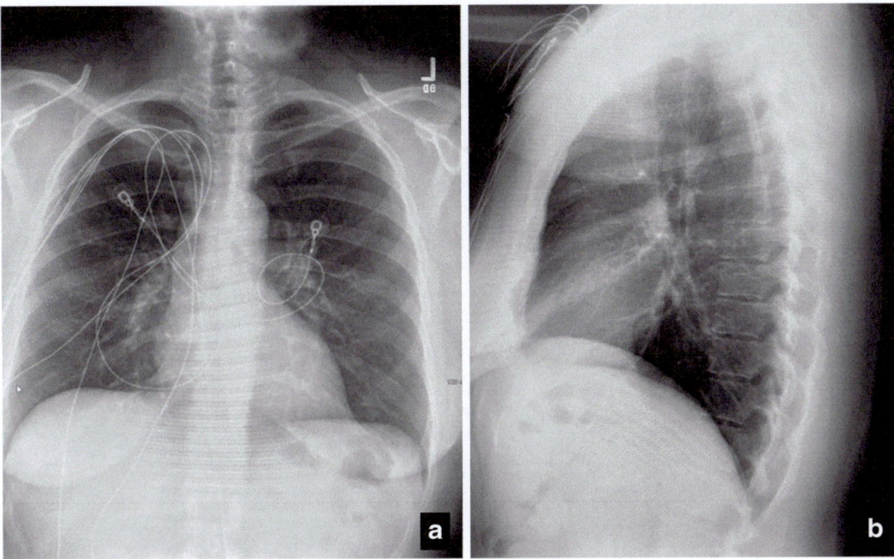

Fig. 8.2 Chest radiograph (CXR) posteroanterior(**a**) and lateral (**b**): Vascular congestion. (Author's own image)

Table 8.1 Complete blood count

Complete blood count	
White blood cells	11×10^9/L
Hemoglobin	10 g/dL
Hematocrit	30%
Platelets	90×110^9/L

Table 8.2 Comprehensive metabolic panel

Comprehensive metabolic panel	
Sodium	136 mEq/L
Potassium	3.9 mEq/L
Chloride	104 mEq/L
Bicarbonate	24 mEq/L
Glucose	96 mg/dL
Blood urea nitrogen (BUN)	52 mg/dL
Creatinine	2.1 mg/dL
Calcium	8.8 mg/dL
Total bilirubin	1.0 mg/dL
Alkaline phosphatase	200 units/L
Aspartate aminotransferase (AST)	120 units/L
Alanine aminotransferase (ALT)	140 units/L
Albumin	4.0 g/dL
Total protein	6.0 g/dL

Table 8.3 Venous blood gas and lactic acid

Venous blood gas and lactic acid	
pH	7.38
pCO2	40 mmHg
pO2	98 mmHg
HCO3	24 mEq/L
Lactic acid	2.2 mEq/L

Table 8.4 Coagulopathy panel

Coagulopathy panel	
International normalized ratio (INR)	1.2
Prothrombin time (PT)	18 seconds
Activated partial thromboplastin time (aPTT)	45 seconds

Table 8.5 Urine dipstick

Urinalysis	
Color	Yellow
Appearance	Foamy
Specific gravity	1.010
pH	6.5
Glucose	1+
Bilirubin	Negative
Ketones	Negative
Protein	3+
Leukocyte esterase	Negative
Nitrites	Negative
White blood cells (WBCs)	Negative
Red blood cells (RBCs)	Negative

Table 8.6 Serum lactate dehydrogenase (LDH)

LDH	390 IU/L

Table 8.7 Serum uric acid

Uric acid	8 mg/dL

Learning Points

Background

Eclampsia is a pregnancy-related hypertensive emergency characterized by the presence of a seizure in a patient with preeclampsia. Other types of pregnancy-related hypertensive disorders include chronic hypertension, gestational hypertension, and preeclampsia. Preeclampsia is defined as a blood pressure ≥ 140/90 at least two times, measured more than 4 hours apart, or ≥ 160/110 sustained over 15 minutes, in a previously normotensive patient who is more than 20 weeks gestation or less than 6 weeks postpartum [1].

The current understanding of the pathophysiology of preeclampsia is that abnormal remodeling of the vessels of the placenta due to an oversupply of cytotrophoblasts leads to ischemia and a change in vasculature of not only the endometrium, but also multiple organ systems due to a cascade of free radicals and cytokines [2]. Hemolysis, elevated liver enzymes, low platelets (HELLP) syndrome was once considered a complication of preeclampsia, but more recently, this concept has been challenged. HELLP syndrome is now considered its own condition, which happens to be frequently associated with hypertension [3]. Eclampsia, specifically, is caused by hypertension resulting in changes in the function and regulation of cerebral vessels, leading to compromised perfusion of the brain and ultimately generalized tonic-clonic seizures.

Risk factors for eclampsia include maternal comorbidities (gestational diabetes, chronic hypertension, chronic kidney disease), advanced maternal age, nulliparity, multiple gestation, obesity, African American or Hispanic race and ethnicity, lower socioeconomic status, and assisted reproductive technology [1, 4].

Early recognition and intervention for preeclampsia and eclampsia are paramount in initiating therapeutic management, to ensure a safe and healthy outcome for both expectant parent and fetus, or the recently postpartum patient.

Differential Diagnosis HELLP (hemolysis, elevated liver enzymes, low platelets) syndrome, postpartum hemorrhage, amniotic fluid embolus, uterine rupture.

History and Physical Exam

The most important historical elements when considering eclampsia or preeclampsia include the prenatal course and gestational age, and whether the patient is postpartum. Eclampsia can be diagnosed up to 6 weeks postpartum. The patient should describe whether there was any prodromal symptoms (e.g., headache, vision change, paresthesia, shortness of breath, nausea, vomiting, and/or abdominal pain) [1]. Any bystanders present should describe the seizure activity appearance and duration as well as any postictal state.

Physical exam should evaluate for complications of hypertension, traumatic injury secondary to seizure, or complications of bleeding due to HELLP syndrome. Elevated blood pressure is necessary for a diagnosis of preeclampsia. Gestational hypertension, the diagnosis of hypertension (systolic blood pressure $\geq$ 140 mmHg and/or diastolic blood pressure $\geq$ 90 mmHg with previously normal blood pressure) after 20 weeks gestation can lead to preeclampsia.

Laboratory Studies

With elevated blood pressure, a patient can also have proteinuria, liver dysfunction, renal dysfunction, pulmonary congestion, central nervous dysfunction, and/or thrombocytopenia. Proteinuria is defined as a protein to creatinine ratio of $\geq$0.3 mg/

dL or 300 mg of protein in urine collected over a 24-hour period. However, proteinuria is no longer mandatory for the diagnosis of preeclampsia and eclampsia [5].

Laboratory studies that indicate end organ damage and/or hemolysis may indicate severe preeclampsia or impending eclampsia [6]. A complete blood count should evaluate for acute anemia or thrombocytopenia. A complete metabolic profile can evaluate for acute kidney injury. Elevated transaminases greater than twice the upper limit of normal, suggests hepatic injury. A disseminated intravascular coagulopathy (DIC) panel can be considered to evaluate for hemolysis (fibrinogen, D-dimer, fibrin split products, prolonged prothrombin time, and international normalized ratio (INR)). Elevated levels of lactate dehydrogenase and uric acid can also indicate hemolysis.

Imaging Findings

There are no specific imaging findings that will confirm the diagnosis of preeclampsia or eclampsia.

If the patient is antepartum and otherwise stable, the fetus should be evaluated by an ultrasound and/or cardiotocographic monitoring. In the ED, point-of-care ultrasound can help confirm that there is a viable fetus by assessing for fetal movement and the fetal heart rate.

Once the patient is stabilized, computed tomography (CT) of the head without contrast can be performed to evaluate for other anatomic lesions in the brain (e.g., cerebral edema, infarction, or hemorrhage) that can cause seizures. When a lesion is identified with eclampsia, the parietal and occipital lobes are commonly involved [6, 7]. In severe preeclampsia and eclampsia, chest radiographs may show signs of pulmonary edema.

Management

Delivery is the ultimate treatment for preeclampsia and eclampsia [8, 9]. In the acute setting of a patient with eclampsia, the immediate response is to stabilize the patient according to the primary survey (airway, breathing, and circulation). According to the primary survey, the eclamptic seizures should be the next priority for intervention. Timely intervention affords the best outcomes for both the mother and the fetus. Magnesium is the mainstay intervention for eclamptic seizures. The initial loading dose of magnesium sulfate is 4–6 grams given parenterally over 15 minutes, followed by a continuous infusion of 1–2 grams per hour for 24 hours or until 24 hours after delivery, whichever lasts longer. Notably, these are high levels of intravascular magnesium and therefore it is important to closely monitor the mother for signs of magnesium toxicity: respiratory depression, central nervous depression, and/or muscle weakness. One of the most accessible bedside markers is

Table 8.8 Antihypertensive dosing for preeclampsia and eclampsia

Labetalol	20 mg IV, doubled every 10 minutes until target blood pressure is achieved, up to 80 mg (300 mg cumulative)
	i.e., 20 mg, then 40 mg, then 80 mg, then 80 mg, then 80 mg
	Or
	1–8 mg/minute infusion
Nifedipine	10 mg oral
	Can be repeated at 30 minutes from first dose at 20 mg oral
	Can be repeated at 60 minutes from first dose at 20 mg oral
Hydralazine	10–20 mg IV every 2–4 hours

the finding of depressed peripheral reflexes. Serum magnesium levels and renal function can also aid in the evaluation for hypermagnesemia. If symptomatic hypermagnesemia develops, the antidote of choice for magnesium toxicity is parenteral calcium.

If seizures continue despite magnesium infusion, antiepileptics are indicated. Benzodiazepines or barbiturates are the antiepileptic drugs of choice.

Magnesium infusion will act as a mild antihypertensive, but ultimately, most patients will require targeted drugs for this hypertensive emergency (Table 8.8). Treatment should begin within 30–60 minutes of recognition of the disease. Parenteral labetalol and hydralazine are preferred first-line agents for acutely ill patients. Oral nifedipine may be an option for the more stable patient.

There are no best practices for the ideal rate of blood pressure correction in preeclampsia. However, the general consensus is to reduce the systolic blood pressure by approximately 25% in the first hour (especially if systolic blood pressure is >200 mmHg). In patients with severe preeclampsia, a generally accepted blood pressure goal is 160/110 mmHg within the first few hours, then 110–140/70–85 mmHg for maintenance [10].

Corticosteroids should be given to the antepartum patient with fetus less than 34 weeks gestational age in anticipation of premature delivery, to facilitate fetal lung development [11].

Consultation Considerations

Obstetrics should be consulted early when preeclampsia or eclampsia is suspected [11]. This is especially critical in the antepartum period when the definitive management is delivery of the fetus, regardless of gestational age. The method of delivery will be determined by the obstetrician based on optimizing both maternal and fetal factors. For the postpartum patient, obstetricians will typically lead the efforts in optimizing the patient's blood pressure and prevention of subsequent seizures. Cardiology or neurology consultations are rarely indicated.

Emergency Department Course and Outcome

As the patient care technician placed the patient on the cardiac monitor in the ED, the patient's eyes started to roll backwards with an upward deviation, and her body started to convulse. The physician requested the nurse to administer a *stat* dose of magnesium sulfate 4 g over 15 minutes. The patient's seizures stopped after approximately 5 minutes. Her repeat blood pressure measurement was 220/109 mmHg. The physician ordered a continuous infusion of labetalol starting at 1 mg/min with repeat blood pressure measurements every 10 minutes until a systolic blood pressure of 140 mmHg and/or diastolic blood pressure of 100 mmHg was achieved. The physician consulted the obstetrics team with a request for admission for further monitoring and management of eclampsia.

The patient received a magnesium infusion for 24 hours and received continuous evaluation, monitoring, and antihypertensive management. She was ultimately discharged from the hospital 4 days later with a prescription to take a daily aspirin and oral labetalol tablets. Her discharge instructions included outpatient follow-up with obstetrics and gynecology in 1 week for repeat laboratory tests and reassessment.

Key Points

- Eclampsia is a pregnancy-related hypertensive disorder characterized by seizures in patients who are more than 20 weeks gestation or less than 6 weeks postpartum, without a prior history of hypertension or epilepsy.
- Symptoms of severe preeclampsia that may precede eclampsia include confusion, headache, changes in vision, shortness of breath, nausea, vomiting, abdominal pain, and/or peripheral edema.
- Management of eclampsia includes immediate delivery of the fetus, a loading dose of magnesium 4–6 grams followed by a continuous infusion, and antihypertensives.

References

1. Gestational Hypertension and Preeclampsia. ACOG practice bulletin, number 222. Obstet Gynecol. 2020;135(6):e237–60. https://doi.org/10.1097/aog.0000000000003891.
2. Magley M, Hinson MR. Eclampsia. In: StatPearls [internet]. Treasure Island: StatPearls Publishing; 2022. Available from: https://www.ncbi.nlm.nih.gov/books/NBK554392/
3. Fitzpatrick KE, Hinshaw K, Kurinczuk JJ, Knight M. Risk factors, management, and outcomes of hemolysis, elevated liver enzymes, and low platelets syndrome and elevated liver enzymes, low platelets syndrome. Obstet Gynecol. 2014;123(3):618–27.
4. Wheeler SM, Myers SO, Swamy GK, Myers ER. Estimated prevalence of risk factors for preeclampsia among individuals giving birth in the US in 2019. JAMA Netw Open. 2022;5(1):e2142343. https://doi.org/10.1001/jamanetworkopen.2021.42343.
5. Fishel Bartal M, Lindheimer MD, Sibai BM. Proteinuria during pregnancy: definition, pathophysiology, methodology, and clinical significance. Am J Obstet Gynecol. 2022;226(2S):S819–34. https://doi.org/10.1016/j.ajog.2020.08.108.

6. FitzGerald MP, Floro C, Siegel J, Hernandez E. Laboratory findings in hypertensive disorders of pregnancy. J Natl Med Assoc. 1996;88(12):794–8.
7. Gurjar B, Rawat RP. CT scan findings in patients of eclampsia. Int J Reprod Contracept Obstet Gynecol. 2017;6(8):3405–8. https://doi.org/10.18203/2320-1770.ijrcog20173452.
8. Wagner LK. Diagnosis and management of preeclampsia. Am Fam Physician. 2004;70(12):2317–24.
9. Wiles K, Damodaram M, Frise C. Severe hypertension in pregnancy. Clin Med (Lond). 2021;21(5):e451–6. https://doi.org/10.7861/clinmed.2021-0508.
10. Brown MA, Magee LA, Kenny LC, et al. International Society for the Study of hypertension in pregnancy (ISSHP). Hypertensive disorders of pregnancy: ISSHP classification, diagnosis, and management recommendations for international practice. Hypertension. 2018;72:24–43.
11. Karrar SA, Hong PL. Preeclampsia. In: StatPearls [internet]. Treasure Island (FL): StatPearls Publishing; 2022. Available from: https://www.ncbi.nlm.nih.gov/books/NBK570611/

Thromboembolic Disease in Pregnancy

9

Coagulation! You're Going to Be a Mom!

Sadia Jamshad and Adeola A. Kosoko

Case

A 32-year-old woman, G3P2 at 36 weeks' gestation, with history of hypertension and hyperlipidemia, presents to the emergency department (ED) with dyspnea on exertion and associated chest pain that is worse with inspiration. She explains that she used to be able to walk a mile without issue, but this past week she has only been walking half of her usual distance due to feeling short of breath. About one week ago, she also noticed her right lower leg appeared more swollen than the left, but she attributed the finding to "normal" pregnancy changes.

- Past medical history: Obesity (body mass index of 33), hypertension, hyperlipidemia
- Past surgical history: None
- Medications: Prenatal vitamins, ferrous sulfate, over-the-counter probiotic supplements, lisinopril
- Allergies: No known drug allergies

Supplementary Information The online version contains supplementary material available at https://doi.org/10.1007/978-3-031-70118-4_9.

S. Jamshad · A. A. Kosoko (✉)
Department of Emergency Medicine, McGovern School of Medicine, University of Texas Health Sciences Center at Houston, Houston, TX, USA
e-mail: Adeola.A.Kosoko@uth.tmc.edu

- Family history: Mother with hypertension
- Social history: Cigarette smoker from ages 17 to 25. Denies alcohol use. Denies illicit drug use.

Physical Exam

- Vital signs
  - Heart rate: 132 beats/minute
  - Blood pressure: 124/78 mmHg
  - Respiratory rate: 24 breaths/minute
  - Temperature: 99 °F
  - Oxygen saturation: 94% on room air
- General appearance: Alert, in mild respiratory distress
- HEENT
  - Head: Normocephalic, atraumatic
  - Eyes: Pupils equal and reactive to light, extraocular movements intact
  - Ears: Normal external ear, normal tympanic membranes
  - Nose: Patent nares
  - Throat: No posterior pharyngeal erythema
  - Neck: Supple, trachea midline, no stridor
- Heart: Tachycardia, no murmur, 2+ distal pulses
- Lungs: Increased work of breathing (pausing in between sentences), lungs clear to auscultation bilaterally, no wheezing, no crackles
- Abdominal/GI: Soft, nontender, nondistended
- Genitourinary: Normal external genitalia, no vaginal bleeding or loss of fluids. Internal exam deferred.
- Extremities: Bilateral lower extremity edema, right leg larger than left leg. Tenderness to palpation at the right inguinal area
- Back: Normal
- Neuro: Alert and oriented x 3. No focal deficits.
- Skin: Warm, dry, no rashes, no cyanosis
- Psych: Normal

Pertinent Diagnostic Tests (Figs. 9.1, 9.2, 9.3 and 9.4, Tables 9.1, 9.2, 9.3, 9.4, 9.5, 9.6 and 9.7)

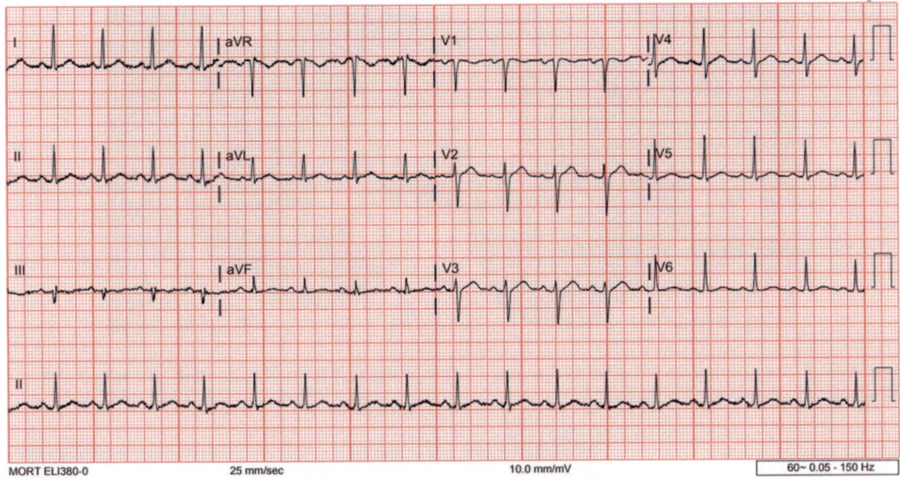

Fig. 9.1 Electrocardiogram (ECG): Normal sinus rhythm. Normal axis/intervals. No obvious signs of ischemia. (S. Jamshad's own image)

Fig. 9.2 Chest radiograph (CXR): No acute abnormality. Cardiac silhouette within normal limits. (S. Jamshad's own image)

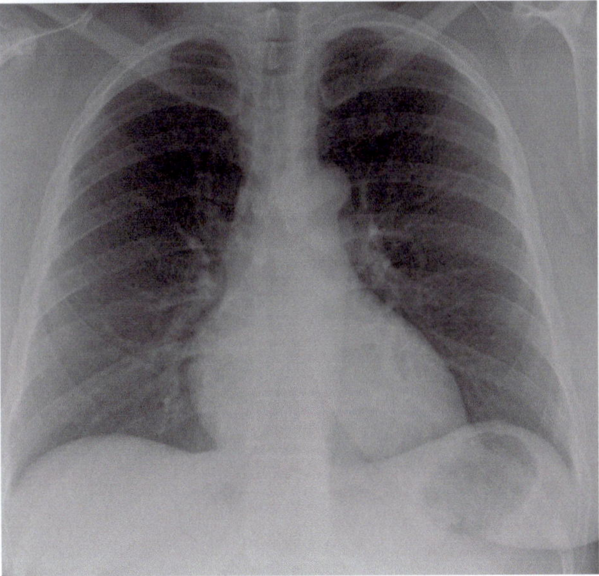

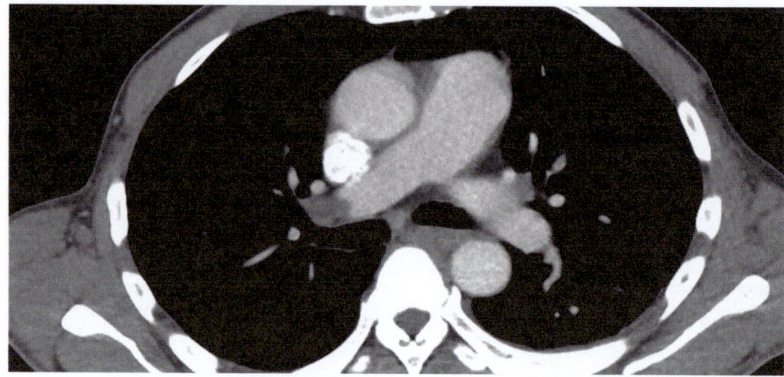

Fig. 9.3 Computed tomographic pulmonary angiogram (CTPA): Right main pulmonary artery embolus. (S. Jamshad's own image)

Fig. 9.4 Doppler ultrasound right lower extremity (DUS RLE): Inability to completely compress common femoral vein. (Images courtesy of Rachel Bower, MD)

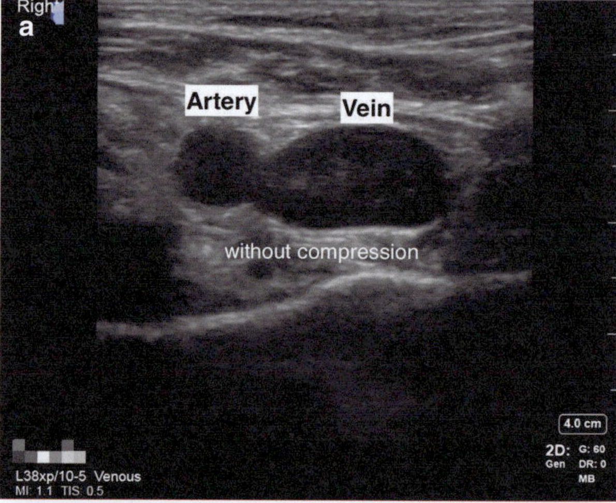

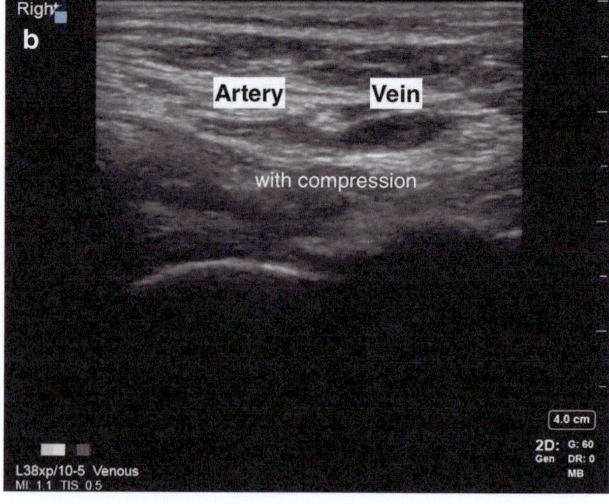

Table 9.1   Complete blood count

Complete blood count	
White blood cells	7.7×10^9/L
Hemoglobin	11.0 g/dL
Hematocrit	40.8%
Platelets	225×10^9/L

Table 9.2   Comprehensive metabolic panel

Comprehensive metabolic panel	
Sodium	138 mEq/L
Potassium	3.8 mEq/L
Chloride	105 mEq/L
Bicarbonate	25 mEq/L
Glucose	92 mg/dL
Blood urea nitrogen (BUN)	11 mg/dL
Creatinine	0.6 mg/dL
Calcium	9.4 mg/dL
Total bilirubin	0.5 mg/dL
Alkaline phosphatase	68 units/L
Aspartate aminotransferase (AST)	20 units/L
Alanine aminotransferase (ALT)	22 units/L
Albumin	3.8 g/dL
Total protein	7.0 g/dL

Table 9.3   Venous blood gas and lactic acid

Venous blood gas and lactic acid	
pH	7.42
pCO2	35 mmHg
pO2	68 mmHg
HCO3	20 mEq/L
Lactic acid	1.1 mEq/L

Table 9.4   D-dimer

D-dimer	
D-dimer	1020 ng/mL

Table 9.5   Troponin

Troponin	
Troponin	<0.03 ng/mL

Table 9.6   Coagulopathy panel

Coagulopathy panel	
International normalized ratio (INR)	1.1
Prothrombin time (PT)	13.6 seconds
Activated partial thromboplastin time (aPTT)	33.5 seconds

Table 9.7 Urinalysis

Urinalysis	
Color	Yellow
Appearance	Clear
Specific gravity	1.011
pH	6.0
Glucose	Negative
Bilirubin	Negative
Ketones	Trace
Protein	Negative
Leukocyte esterase	Negative
Nitrites	Negative
White blood cells (WBC)	2 WBCs/high-power field (HPF)
Red blood cells (RBC)	0 RBCs/HPF
Squamous epithelial cells	2 Cells/HPF

Learning Points

Background

Thromboembolic disease occurs when clotted blood obstructs a blood vessel. Mortality is dependent on the size, location, and acuity of the obstruction. It can occur in any organ system and therefore, depending on the organ involved, presentation will vary. The most described thromboembolisms in pregnant patients occur in the form of pulmonary embolism (PE) or deep vein thrombosis (DVT). Thromboembolic disease in pregnancy is the leading cause of morbidity and mortality in this patient population [1]. The pregnant state induces an intrinsic hypercoagulable state, making these patients at a high risk for venous thromboembolism (VTE). Therefore, it is imperative for providers to keep a high index of suspicion to recognize and manage these conditions.

The risk of VTE in pregnant women is higher than the general population, starting from conception and including the postpartum period. The highest risk is in the third trimester and the first week postpartum. As with nonpregnant individuals, those with a history of thrombotic events or history of thrombophilia have an elevated risk [1].

Differential Diagnosis Congestive heart failure (CHF), peripartum cardiomyopathy, air embolism or amniotic fluid embolism, pneumonia, acute coronary syndrome (ACS), pre-eclampsia, expected pregnancy changes.

History and Physical Exam

The clinical signs and symptoms of VTE will vary based on the location, size, extent, and acuity of the thrombus. Small, non-occlusive thrombi may be asymptomatic. Large, occlusive thrombi may present with pain, swelling, fever, necrosis, or organ failure, depending on the organ involved.

A pregnant patient or a nonpregnant patient may present with a history and physical exam that includes unilateral extremity swelling, pain, or erythema, suggesting a DVT. Pain is often localized to the calf or the thigh of the lower extremity. Upper extremity DVTs are less common but would present similarly. A patient with a PE may have a history and physical of dyspnea, chest pain, cough, syncope, fatigue, or tachycardia [2].

A thorough history should describe the onset and location of symptoms. The patient should describe current and prior obstetric history. Also, each patient with suspected VTE should be explicitly questioned whether they have had a past diagnosis of VTE and whether the cause was identified. Other risk factors for VTE should be considered in questioning: Any recent major operative procedures? Family history of clotting problems? Any cancer history?

Each patient should have a full set of vital signs documented. Tachycardia can often be one of the first findings by which to consider PE. Of note, two-thirds of pregnant and postpartum women with PEs have a normal oxygen saturation on presentation [3].

Overall, it can be difficult to differentiate between the normal physiologic changes of pregnancy and the presenting signs and symptoms of a PE and DVT, as there is significant overlap between the conditions. The growing uterus typically displaces intra-abdominal organs leading to decreased space for lung expansion, often resulting in shortness of breath in a normal pregnancy. A growing uterus can also cause some compression of the venous structures in the lower abdomen and pelvis causing decreased venous return to the heart, which can lead to lower extremity swelling/edema.

Common clinical risk-stratification tools for DVTs and PEs are the Wells' Criteria or the Pulmonary Embolism Rule-Out Criteria (PERC). However, these tools were not developed nor validated for use in the pregnant population.

Laboratory Studies

A serum D-dimer measurement evaluates for a by-product of fibrinolysis. D-dimer is typically a very *sensitive* blood test to rule out VTE. However, D-dimer is not a *specific* test for VTE because it can be positive in many other conditions, even in a normal pregnancy. Therefore, it is not a good test to rule-in VTE in the low-risk population. A negative D-dimer in any population, however, generally reliably rules out a clinically significant VTE in any low-risk patient. Therefore, when a D-dimer is not elevated in a low-risk patient, VTE is unlikely and confirmatory testing by imaging and empiric anticoagulation are unnecessary. Unfortunately, in the state of pregnancy, even in normal pregnancy, D-dimer is often elevated, often making it a less useful screening tool.

The pregnancy-adapted YEARS clinical criteria algorithm (Fig. 9.5) was crafted to utilize D-dimer more appropriately for screening low-risk pregnant patients who could have a PE. When no YEARS criteria are met and a serum D-dimer <1000 ng/mL, or if a patient has 1–3 of the YEARS criteria and a D-dimer <500 ng/mL, a PE is highly unlikely, and imaging or anticoagulation is unnecessary [4].

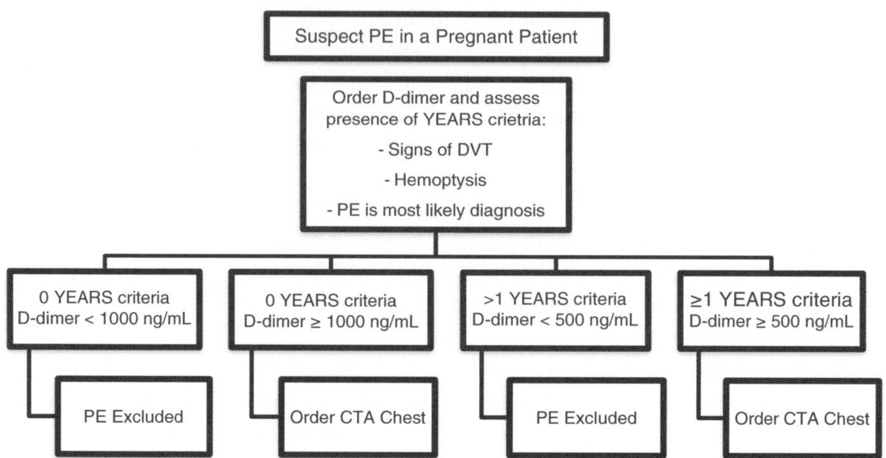

Fig. 9.5 YEARS criteria for suspected PE in a pregnant patient

Other laboratory tests that should be obtained when VTE is suspected include a complete blood count and a coagulation profile.

Imaging Findings

The gold standard for the diagnosis of a DVT is a compression Doppler ultrasound (Duplex US) in both pregnant and nonpregnant patients. Diagnosis with Duplex US is made by visualizing a noncompressible vein based on two-point compression at the highest probability points for identifying a DVT in the deep branches of the veins. Interestingly, DVTs in pregnant patients are more commonly diagnosed on the left side and located in the iliofemoral and iliac veins, whereas in the general population, DVTs are more typically identified in the more distal veins [5]. When there is increased concern for potential proximal VTEs in some pregnant patients with high clinical suspicion but a normal or indeterminant Duplex US, a non-contrast MRI or venogram may be considered to definitively determine whether there is indeed a VTE and how proximal it is progressing. However, data for use of these imaging modalities in the pregnant population is limited [6].

To diagnose a PE, the two most-utilized imaging modalities are the computed tomographic pulmonary angiogram (CTPA) and ventilation/perfusion imaging (V/Q scan). The CTPA can potentially visualize the clot in the pulmonary vasculature, and the V/Q scan can assess if there is a ventilation-perfusion mismatch in the lungs that may be caused by a clot. The CTPA chest has become the gold standard for diagnosis of PE in an emergency setting. In pregnancy, the risk of radiation exposure associated with CTPA, and its effects on the fetus (such as congenital abnormalities, intellectual disability, and childhood cancers), frequently becomes a topic of concern. However, current CTPA protocols utilize radiation levels which are well below the dose levels that significantly increase the risk for congenital abnormalities regardless of gestational age [7]. It is estimated that during the course of gestation, a fetus will be exposed to 1 mGy of baseline background radiation without medical imaging. It is estimated that a CTPA will deliver approximately 0.01–0.66 mGy of radiation per scan. The lowest estimated threshold dose that can result in fetal abnormalities varies by gestational age, but on average appears to be 50 mGy, according to an article from the American College of Obstetricians and Gynecologists [8]. Regardless, *all patients should still be counselled* on general radiation risks and benefits of any imaging. Echocardiography is typically obtained when a pulmonary embolism is identified to determine whether right heart strain is evident, which may require more aggressive interventions (Fig. 9.6).

The V/Q scan, a nuclear medicine test, is also an option to diagnose PE. V/Q scans are particularly useful if the patient is high risk for a PE but has a contraindication to or refuses a CTPA (e.g., a life-threatening intravenous contrast allergy or significant renal failure). V/Q scans, however, lose accuracy in patients with chronic lung disease in those or who may have acutely abnormal chest radiographs.

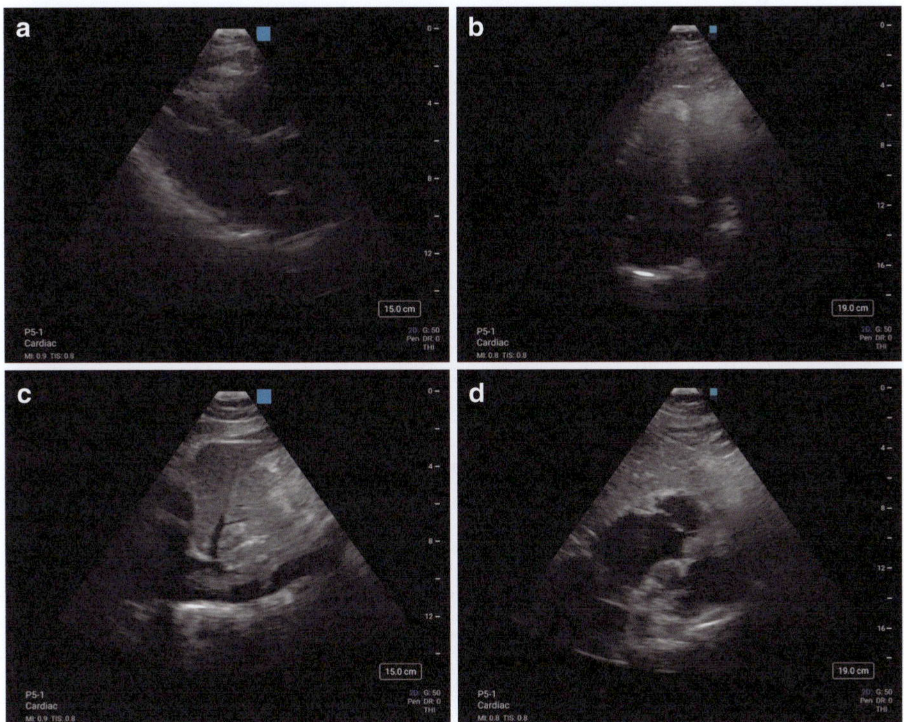

Fig. 9.6 Point-of-Care Cardiac Ultrasound (echocardiogram) (**a**) Parasternal long view, (**b**) Apical four-chamber view, (**c**) Inferior vena cava view, (**d**) Subxiphoid view: Right heart strain and blood clot

Management

The individualized-approach treatment of thromboembolism can be quite complex depending on multiple factors including the size of the vessel involved, the underlying cause of the thrombus, and the patient's hemodynamic status. However, the mainstay of initial management of DVT and PE in the emergency setting during pregnancy is therapeutic anticoagulation. The preferred agents are heparin compounds including unfractionated heparin or low-molecular weight heparin (LMWH) as neither cross the placenta [1]. The American Society of Hematology recommends LMWH over UFH [9]. Warfarin is contraindicated due to its teratogenic effects on the fetus. Oral direct thrombin inhibitors (e.g., dabigatran) and anti-Xa inhibitors (e.g., rivaroxaban, apixaban) should be avoided at this time due to insufficient data on their safety profile in pregnancy [1].

There is limited evidence for the use of systemic or targeted thrombolytics in pregnant patients with massive and sub-massive PEs. These thrombolytics can potentially be administered, if necessary, especially in cases of hemodynamic compromise. Consideration should be made for close monitoring for resultant major bleeding, including uterine bleeding [10].

There is no literature that demonstrates a preference for inpatient or outpatient regimens for management of pregnant patients, in particular, who have low-risk VTEs [11]. Therefore, clinicians should use judgment and assess the patient's entire clinical and social picture when determining hospital admission versus emergency department discharge.

Consultation Considerations

Obstetric teams should be consulted early in the care of a pregnant patient with thromboembolic disease, to provide concurrent fetal monitoring (if indicated), to provide help with possible emergent obstetric complications, and to ensure continuity of inpatient and outpatient care. Obstetricians may also provide guidance on anticoagulation therapies.

In patients who have either a massive or sub-massive PE, interventional cardiologists/pulmonologists or critical care intensivists can be consulted for help managing the hemodynamically unstable patient.

Radiologists may be helpful in recommending imaging modalities and interpreting imaging in the diagnosis of a VTE. An interventional radiologist may be able to perform catheter-directed thrombolysis of a high-grade PE or for placement of an inferior vena cava filter if indicated.

A hematology consultant can assist in the patient's evaluation to decipher whether, aside from pregnancy, there is an underlying pathology (e.g., genetic) which may be further predisposing the patient to thromboembolism. They can also assist in optimizing care for the patient.

Emergency Department Course and Outcome

The patient was placed on 2 liters of oxygen by nasal cannula. She consented to a Doppler ultrasound study of her lower extremity which showed a partially occlusive popliteal DVT. The patient was deemed high risk for a PE and she consented to a CTPA. A left-sided segmental PE was found, and she was started on a heparin infusion. Right heart strain was absent based on the CTPA.

She was admitted to the hospital for further management, with the obstetrics team consulted, due to her oxygen requirement and for general monitoring. Inpatient, she was placed on continuous fetal monitoring which was unremarkable. An echocardiogram lacked right heart strain, pericardial effusion, or any signs of left heart strain. A hematology consultant evaluated the patient and ultimately discovered with further testing that she had a diagnosis of Factor V Leiden, predisposing her to thromboembolic disease. The patient remained hemodynamically stable. In preparation for her discharge home, she transitioned from the heparin drip to therapeutic-dose LMWH every 12 hours. After a 3-day hospital stay, she was discharged home on LMWH with outpatient appointments with her obstetrician and new hematologist.

Key Points

- Signs and symptoms of thromboembolic disease in pregnancy can present similarly to expected changes of pregnancy.
- Doppler ultrasound and computed tomographic pulmonary angiogram are the imaging modalities of choice if suspecting a DVT or PE, even in a pregnant patient.
- Intravenous or subcutaneous therapeutic anticoagulation modalities are the mainstays of treatment for DVTs and PEs (i.e., low molecular weight heparin or unfractionated heparin).

References

1. ACOG practice bulletin no. 196: thromboembolism in pregnancy. Obstet Gynecol 132(1):e1–e17; 2018. 10.1097/AOG.0000000000002706.
2. Goodacre S, Horspool K, Nelson-Piercy C, Knight M, Shephard N, Lecky F, Thomas S, Hunt BJ, Fuller G. The DiPEP study: an observational study of the diagnostic accuracy of clinical assessment, D-dimer and chest x-ray for suspected pulmonary embolism in pregnancy and postpartum. BJOG. 2029;126(3):383–92. https://doi.org/10.1111/s1471052815286.
3. Elgendi IY, Fogerty A, Blanco-Molina A, Rosa V, Schellong S, Skride A, Portillo J, Lopez-Miguel P, Monreal M, Weinberg I. Clinical presentation and outcomes of women presenting with venous thromboembolism during pregnancy and postpartum period: findings from REITE registry. Thrombosis Haemostatis. 2020;120(10):1454–62. https://doi.org/10.1055/s00401714211.

4. van der Pol LM, Tromeur C, Bistervels IM, Ni Ainle F, van Bemmel T, Bertoletti L, Couturaud F, van Dooren YPA, Elias A, Faber LM, Hofstee HMA, van der Hulle T, Kruip MJHA, Maignan M, Mairuhu ATA, Middeldorp S, Nijkeuter M, Roy PM, Sanchez O, Schmidt J, Ten Wolde M, Klok FA, Huisman MV, Artemis Study Investigators. Pregnancy-adapted YEARS algorithm for diagnosis of suspected pulmonary embolism. N Engl J Med. 2019;380(12):1139–49. https://doi.org/10.1056/NEJMoa1813865.
5. Chan WS, Spencer FA, Ginsberg JS. Anatomic distribution of deep vein thrombosis in pregnancy. CMAJ. 2010;182(7):657–60. https://doi.org/10.1503/cmaj.091692.
6. Spritzer CE, Evans AC, Kay HH. Magnetic resonance imaging of deep venous thrombosis in pregnant women with lower extremity edema. Obstet Gynecol. 1995;85(4):603–7.
7. Schaefer-Prokop C, Prokop M. CTPA for the diagnosis of acute pulmonary embolism during pregnancy. Eur Radiol. 2008;18:2705–8. https://doi.org/10.1007/s00330-008-1158-8.
8. Copel J, et al. Guidelines for diagnostic imaging during pregnancy and lactation committee opinion No. 723. American College of Obstetrics and Gynecologists. Obstet Gynecol. 2017;130:e210–6.
9. Schünemann HJ, Cushman M, Burnett AE, Kahn SR, Beyer-Westendorf J, Spencer FA, Rezende SM, Zakai NA, Bauer KA, Dentali F, Lansing J, Balduzzi S, Darzi A, Morgano GP, Neumann I, Nieuwlaat R, Yepes-Nuñez JJ, Zhang Y, Wiercioch W. American Society of Hematology 2018 guidelines for management of venous thromboembolism: prophylaxis for hospitalized and nonhospitalized medical patients. Blood Adv. 2018;2(22):3198–225. https://doi.org/10.1182/bloodadvances.2018022954.
10. Rodriguez D, Jerjes-Sanchez C, Fonseca S, et al. Thrombolysis in massive and submassive pulmonary embolism during pregnancy and the puerperium: a systematic review. J Thromb Thrombolysis. 2020;50:929–41. https://doi.org/10.1007/s11239-020-02122-7.
11. Bates SM, Rajasekhar A, Middeldorp S, McLintock C, Rodger MA, James AH, Vazquesz SR, Greer IA, Riva JJ, Bhatt M, Schwab N, Barrett D, LaHaye A, Rochwerg B. American Society of Hematology 2018 guidelines for management of venous thromboembolism: venous thromboembolism in the context of pregnancy. Blood Adv. 2018;2(22):3317–59. https://doi.org/10.1182/bloodadvanves.2018024802.

Premature Rupture of Membranes

10

Did I Pee Myself?

Zoë R. Fisher and Adeola A. Kosoko

Case

A 36-year-old woman, G2P1, 37 weeks' gestational age by first trimester ultrasound, presents to the emergency department (ED) for "vaginal leaking" after a low-speed motor vehicle collision (MVC). The MVC was 3 days ago, and she did not seek medical care at that time because she did not have pain and there was minimal damage to the car. She has generally felt normal since then, but she became concerned today when she noticed clear fluid intermittently leaking from her vagina onto her legs, which has continued for the past two hours. She denies any vaginal bleeding, abdominal cramping, pain in her extremities, nausea, or vomiting. She feels the baby moving with the same frequency as before the accident. She has been to all her prenatal appointments and is Group B *Streptococcus* (GBS) negative.

- Past medical history: G2P1 with regular prenatal care, normal prenatal course to date
- Past surgical history: None
- Medications: Prenatal vitamins
- Allergies: No known drug allergies
- Family history: Mother has hypertension
- Social history: No alcohol. Smokes one pack of cigarettes per week. No illicit drug use.

Z. R. Fisher (✉) · A. A. Kosoko
Department of Emergency Medicine, McGovern School of Medicine, University of Texas
Health Sciences Center at Houston, Houston, TX, USA
e-mail: zoe.r.fisher@uth.tmc.edu; Adeola.A.Kosoko@uth.tmc.edu

A. A. Kosoko (ed.), *Emergency Medicine Case-Based Guide*,
https://doi.org/10.1007/978-3-031-70118-4_10

Physical Exam

- Vital signs
  - Heart rate: 85 beats/minute
  - Blood pressure: 118/72 mmHg
  - Respiratory rate: 14 breaths/minute
  - Temperature: 98.7 °F
  - Oxygen saturation: 97% on room air
- General appearance: Appears older than stated age, sitting up in the bed, anxious appearing.
- HEENT
  - Head: Atraumatic, normocephalic
  - Eyes: Pupils equal, round, and reactive to light (4–2 mm); external ocular movements are normal; normal conjunctiva; no papilledema
  - Ears: Normal
  - Nose: Normal
  - Throat: No erythema or edema of the oropharynx
  - Neck: Trachea midline, no stridor, no jugular venous distention
- Heart: Normal rate, regular rhythm, equal pulses
- Lungs: Clear to auscultation bilaterally, no rales or rhonchi
- Abdominal: Soft, nontender, bowel sounds present, gravid with fundus above the umbilicus
- Genitourinary: Normal external, no vaginal bleeding, speculum exam shows cloudy fluid pooling at posterior fornix with open exterior os, bimanual deferred
- Rectal: Normal
- Extremities: 1+ pitting edema at the ankles, no tenderness, no deformity, tolerates full range of motion, negative Homans' sign bilaterally
- Back: Normal
- Neuro: Alert, oriented, normal reflexes, no clonus
- Skin: Normal
- Lymph: Normal
- Psych: Normal

Pertinent Diagnostic Tests (Figs. 10.1 and 10.2, Tables 10.1, 10.2, 10.3, 10.4 and 10.5)

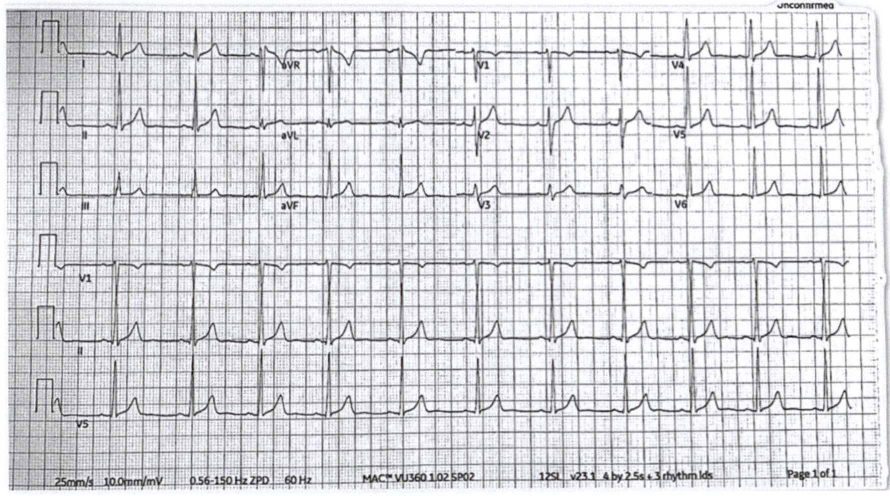

Fig. 10.1 Electrocardiogram (ECG): Normal sinus rhythm. (Z. Fisher's own image)

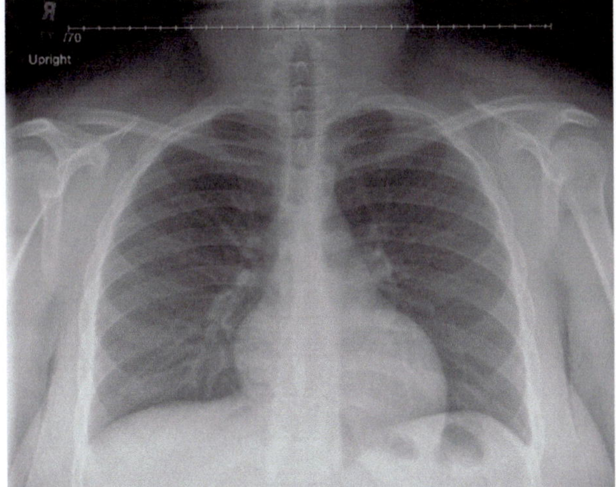

Fig. 10.2 Chest radiograph (CXR): Normal CXR (Z. Fisher's own image)

Table 10.1 Complete blood count

Complete blood count	
White blood cells	14×10^9/L
Hemoglobin	13 g/dL
Hematocrit	30%
Platelets	340×10^9/L

Table 10.2 Comprehensive metabolic panel

Comprehensive metabolic panel	
Sodium	140 mEq/L
Potassium	4.1 mEq/L
Chloride	108 mEq/L
Bicarbonate	26 mEq/L
Glucose	79 mg/dL
Blood urea nitrogen (BUN)	22 mg/dL
Creatinine	0.7 mg/dL
Calcium	9 mg/dL
Total bilirubin	0.6 mg/dL
Alkaline phosphatase	60 units/L
Aspartate aminotransferase (AST)	70 units/L
Alanine aminotransferase (ALT)	100 units/L
Albumin	4.0 g/dL
Total protein	7.2 g/dL

Table 10.3 Venous blood gas and lactic acid

Venous blood gas and lactic acid	
pH	7.40
pCO2	40 mmHg
pO2	108 mmHg
HCO3	20 mEq/L
Lactic acid	0.6 mEq/L

Table 10.4 Coagulopathy panel

Coagulopathy panel	
International normalized ratio (INR)	1.0
Prothrombin time (PT)	12.4 seconds
Activated partial thromboplastin time (aPTT)	23.1 seconds

Table 10.5 Urinalysis

Urinalysis	
Color	Yellow
Appearance	Clear
Specific gravity	1.020
pH	7.1
Glucose	Negative
Bilirubin	Negative
Ketones	0
Protein	1+
Leukocyte esterase	Trace
Nitrites	Negative
White blood cells (WBCs)	0 WBCs/high-power field (HPF)
Red blood cells (RBCs)	0 RBCs/HPF
Squamous epithelial cells	0–5 cells/HPF

Learning Points

Background

Premature rupture of membranes (PROM) is the rupture of the gestational (placenta) membrane leading to the external detection of amniotic fluid *after* 37 weeks gestational age but before active labor. Preterm premature rupture of membranes (PPROM) is the rupture of the gestational (placenta) membrane *before* 37 weeks of gestation, before active labor, and with external detection of amniotic fluid [1]. Patients with PROM are more likely to present to the ED setting.

PROM accounts for about 10% of all pregnancies while PPROM is present in up to one-third of all preterm births [1]. Any rupture of membranes may be due to natural weakening of the membranes expected with the progression of pregnancy; however, PPROM is often due to weakening of the membranes due to infection of the uterus [2].

Risk factors for PROM include but are not limited to prior preterm birth, antepartum bleeding, Black race (non-Hispanic), cervical insufficiency, poly- or oligohydramnios, multiple gestation, cigarette smoking during pregnancy, illicit drug use, sexually transmitted infections, low body mass index, and prior pregnancy with PROM [3].

The diagnosis of PPROM indicates that the baby is likely to be born within a few days of the membrane rupture. PPROM is also linked with the risk of serious infection of the placental tissues, placing both the mother and fetus at risk. A diagnosis of PROM puts the mother and fetus at risk for placental abruption, umbilical cord injury, and postpartum infection. Unfortunately, because many cases of PPROM also have fetal malpresentation, there is an increased risk of cesarean delivery and associated surgical complications [1].

Differential Diagnosis Urinary incontinence, cystocele, vaginal bleeding, vaginal discharge, cervical mucus, placental abruption.

History and Physical Exam

Any woman presenting with a complaint of leakage of fluids should receive a thorough review of all elements of the medical history. Many women may state that they felt that they may have urinated on themselves. Some may explain that they felt their "water break" or a constant moisture in their underwear. They may even describe a feeling of liquid tracking down their legs. Any history describing the presence of potential vaginal fluids should be investigated critically, including timing, quantity of fluids, quality of fluids, any pain, vaginal bleeding, recent sexual activity, traumatic injury, or patterns in contractions or fetal movements.

Determine the gestational age of the fetus. If the patient is unsure, ultrasound is the best means of determining the gestational age. Using the last menstrual period to determine the gestational age is a secondary option. The well-being of the fetus should be evaluated by determining the fetal heart rate either by Doppler auscultation or duplex ultrasound.

A general physical exam should be performed, but the genitourinary evaluation is the most important to diagnose PROM and PPROM. It must be performed in a way that minimizes the risk of infection. Therefore, a sterile speculum exam should be used to evaluate for drainage of amniotic fluid from the cervix or pooling of fluids in the introitus which would suggest rupture of membranes. The speculum exam will also evaluate for any signs of infection, umbilical cord prolapse, fluid collection, bleeding, or fetal prolapse. A digital exam or bimanual exam is generally unnecessary if considering ruptured membranes unless the patient is in active labor. Sterile gloves should be used for the digital exam during suspected active labor and cervical dilatation should be measured. If indicated, cultures can be obtained during the sterile speculum exam.

Laboratory Studies

The traditional diagnosis of rupture of membranes consists of three parts: (1) visualization, on sterile speculum exam, of pooling of clear fluid in the vagina, originating from the cervix; (2) an alkaline pH of the sample obtained of the pooled fluid; and (3) "ferning" of a sample of the pooled fluid [1].

Amniotic fluid is usually more alkaline (pH 7.1–7.3) than normal vaginal secretions, which tend to have a pH ranging from 4.5 to 6.0. However, certain exposures can alter the pH of vaginal fluids, including blood, semen, douching agents, or infection (particularly bacterial vaginosis). A common method is to measure the pH of the fluid sample using pH paper. A specific pH test is the nitrazine test. A nitrazine test strip is yellow at baseline, but upon contact with amniotic fluid (or other alkaline fluid) it will turn blue, indicating that the fluid is basic. Contact with typical vaginal secretions will generally maintain the yellow color of the strip. The nitrazine test is the most common test used to confirm clinical diagnosis of ruptured membranes.

Additionally, one can smear a thin sample of the obtained fluid on a glass slide and observe a resultant pattern resembling a fern plant when the sample has dried and crystallized (Fig. 10.3). This characteristic microscopic finding is called "ferning" or "arborization" and is highly suggestive of an amniotic fluid sample and therefore rupture of membranes.

There are also commercial testing kits that can aid in differentiating amniotic fluid from other fluids. Specifically, these kits tend to measure biomarkers that are characteristically in amniotic fluids (e.g., alpha-fetoprotein, fetal fibronectin, prolactin, beta chorionic gonadotropin (β-hCG), and placental alpha macroglobulin-1 (PAMG-1)). These biomarkers should be absent if membranes are intact and the sample is that of vaginal secretions or other fluids. Fetal fibronectin tests can help determine if fetal membranes have ruptured; however, research shows that its use has not reduced the number of preterm births [4]. An increasingly popular bedside test is the rapid PAMG-1 rapid immunoassay. PAMG-1 is

Fig. 10.3 "Ferning" of an amniotic fluid sample. (Image courtesy of Allyson Rowe, MD, used with permission)

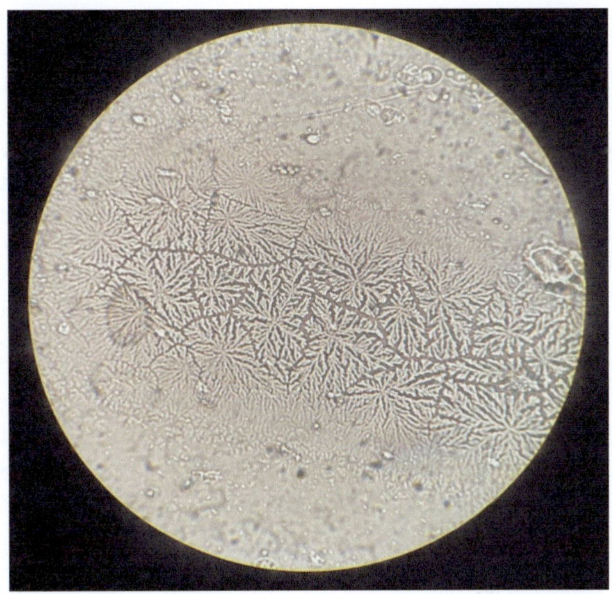

a protein present in amniotic fluid but rare in vaginal fluid or maternal blood. The test can identify even trace amounts of PAMG-1, aiding in diagnosis of PROM with sensitivity of about 99% and specificity of 100% [2]. With such a sensitive and specific test, a sterile speculum exam is not necessary to collect a fluid sample; rather, a less invasive means of obtaining the fluid can be used: a sterile swab can be directly inserted into the vagina, and the assay can produce results in less than 10 minutes.

Imaging Findings

Ultrasound of the uterus and fetus can be performed to evaluate the fetal heart rate and to determine the amniotic fluid index, evaluating for poly- or oligohydramnios. Ultrasound by itself cannot determine ruptured membranes.

Management

The optimal care of a patient with PROM is individualized based on the age of the fetus and the risk of infection.

Early term, term, and late preterm gestational ages (generally all patients 34 weeks' gestation and older) should have the mother receive Group B *Streptococcus* (GBS) prophylaxis if indicated, and the fetus should be delivered.

Preterm gestational ages (24–33 weeks' gestation) should receive GBS prophylaxis if indicated, corticosteroids, antibiotics, and expectant management [5].

At any time, if fetal monitoring is concerning, or if there are signs of chorioamnionitis (i.e., maternal fever, tachycardia, uterine tenderness, or cloudy or colored amniotic fluid), delivery of the fetus should occur. Similarly, if there is vaginal bleeding, it may indicate placental abruption, and the fetus may need emergent delivery [1].

Glucocorticoids (intramuscular betamethasone 12 mg daily for 2 days or intramuscular dexamethasone 6 mg twice daily for 2 days) should be strongly considered if the patient could potentially deliver at 24–34 weeks' gestation. Glucocorticoids may help decrease the risk of fetal health complications, including respiratory distress syndrome, intraventricular hemorrhage, and necrotizing enterocolitis [2]. Benefit from glucocorticoids may be seen from 4 hours of administration and up to 7 days after administration. However, there is no proven benefit to routine glucocorticoid administration after 34 weeks' gestation [1]. Research does not support the use of tocolysis following a diagnosis of PROM after 34 weeks' gestation.

Antibiotics targeting GBS should be administered for all women with imminent preterm delivery (> 34 weeks' gestation) unless there is a negative perineal culture documented after 35 weeks [6]. A popular regimen for GBS prophylaxis is intravenous ampicillin (2 g every 6 hours) and erythromycin (250 mg every 6 hours) for 2 days. The patient can be transitioned to oral antibiotics to complete a 7-day course [5].

Patients diagnosed with PROM or PPROM require admission to the hospital for reassessment for signs of infection and for monitoring of the fetus. Currently, there is no way to reliably predict which pregnancies will develop complications or to ensure that a discharged patient will reliably understand or be able to return to the hospital in a timely fashion should complications arise. Outpatient management of PROM is generally impractical.

Consultation Considerations

An obstetrics consult for fetal heart monitoring should be made early in the patient's presentation.

Delivery of the fetus can typically be induced vaginally if spontaneous labor is not presently occurring or does not imminently occur. However, if there are signs of fetal distress, a cesarean section may be necessary to facilitate delivery. The obstetrician should also be able to guide antibiotic and glucocorticoid recommendations and coordinate general inpatient management.

Emergency Department Course and Outcome

The emergency physician completed a pelvic ultrasound after performing a focused abdominal sonography in trauma exam (FAST) due to the patient's recent MVC. The FAST exam was negative. An intrauterine fetus was identified with a heart rate of 157 beats/minute. Lacking other signs of trauma or indications for further imaging to evaluate for traumatic injury, a sterile pelvic exam investigated the chief complaint. A small volume of clear fluid was found pooling in the introitus, and the patient had a positive nitrazine test.

Concerned for a diagnosis of PROM, obstetrics was consulted for admission. The obstetrics team requested a sample of the fluid to be set aside for biomarker testing and evaluation with microscopy. The obstetrics team explained that they would administer any antibiotic or steroid prophylaxis at the labor and delivery unit, and the patient was transported without incident.

Key Points

- Premature rupture of the membranes occurs due to trauma or intrinsic weakening of the connective tissues of the fetal membranes.
- Testing for the nature of the vaginal fluids can be accomplished by pH paper, nitrazine paper, or specialized testing for biochemical markers.
- The best care practices of PROM are determining the gestational age, confirming the diagnosis, documenting fetal viability, and avoiding infection.

References

1. Practice Bulletin No. 160: Premature rupture of membranes. Obstet Gynecol. 2016;127(1):e39–51. https://doi.org/10.1097/aog.0000000000001266.
2. Tchirikov M, Schlabritz-Loutsevitch N, Maher J, Buchmann J, Naberezhnev Y, Winarno AS, et al. Mid-trimester preterm premature rupture of membranes (PPROM): etiology, diagnosis, classification, international recommendations of treatment options and outcome. J Perinat Med. 2018;46(5):465–88. https://doi.org/10.1515/jpm-2017-0027.
3. Cousins LM, Smok DP, Lovett SM, Poeltler DM. AmniSure placental alpha microglobulin-1 rapid immunoassay versus standard diagnostic methods for detection of rupture of membranes. Am J Perinatol. 2005;22(6):317–20. https://doi.org/10.1055/s-2005-870896.
4. Berghella V, Saccone G. Fetal fibronectin testing for reducing the risk of preterm birth. Cochrane Database Syst Rev. 2019;7(7):CD006843. https://doi.org/10.1002/14651858.CD006843.pub3.
5. Petit C, Deruelle P, Behal H, Rakza T, Balagny S, Subtil D, et al. Preterm premature rupture of membranes: which criteria contraindicate home care management? Acta Obstet Gynecol Scand. 2018;97(12):1499–507. https://doi.org/10.1111/aogs.13433.
6. Morgan JA, Zafar N, Cooper DB. Group B Streptococcus and pregnancy. [Updated 2023 Jul 24]. In: StatPearls [Internet]. Treasure Island: StatPearls Publishing; 2023. Available from: https://www.ncbi.nlm.nih.gov/books/NBK482443/

Peri/Post-Mortem Cesarean Section

Cutting-Edge Emergency Medicine

Carolina Mendoza

Case

A 27-year-old woman, G2P1, at 37 weeks' gestation is brought in by emergency medical services (EMS). She was the driver involved in a high-speed, head-on collision during a motor vehicle accident. The patient was found unresponsive on the scene where she had prolonged extrication efforts lasting 30 minutes. The initial EMS assessment found the patient with a faint pulse and normotensive. They started a peripheral fluid bolus of 1 liter of lactated Ringer's solution. The trauma service was activated upon her arrival at the emergency department (ED) and upon her initial assessment the patient who was once in a guarded state, became pulseless, resulting in cardiac arrest. The emergency team alongside the trauma team began resuscitative efforts including cardiopulmonary resuscitation (CPR). The patient was intubated and received breaths via respiratory bag valve. The local massive transfusion protocol was initiated. Her cardiac rhythm was asystole at minute 4 of continuous resuscitation.

- Past medical history: Second pregnancy (G2P1) with regular prenatal care and a normal prenatal course. Previous pregnancy was unremarkable.
- Past surgical history: Unknown
- Medications: Prenatal vitamins
- Allergies: No known drug allergies
- Family history: Unknown
- Social history: Unknown

C. Mendoza (✉)
Department of Emergency Medicine, University of Maryland School of Medicine, Baltimore, MD, USA

© The Author(s), under exclusive license to Springer Nature Switzerland AG 2024
A. A. Kosoko (ed.), *Emergency Medicine Case-Based Guide*,
https://doi.org/10.1007/978-3-031-70118-4_11

Physical Exam

- EMS pre-arrival vital signs
  - Heart rate: 65 beats/minute
  - Blood pressure: 100/60 mmHg
  - Respiratory rate: 12 breaths/minute
  - Temperature: 98.5°F
  - Oxygen saturation: 97% on room air
- Vital signs on arrival: Asystole
- General appearance: Pale, unresponsive
- HEENT
  - Head: Normocephalic, 2 cm linear laceration to right forehead, hemostatic
  - Eyes: Pupils dilated bilaterally and sluggish to direct light
  - Ears: Normal outer ears, no blood in external canal
  - Nose: No deformity, small amount of dry blood in right nostril
  - Throat: Clear, moist
  - Neck: Cervical collar in place, no midline step-offs
- Heart: Asystole
- Lungs: Clear to auscultation bilaterally; no rales, wheezing, or crackles
- Abdominal/GI: Gravid abdomen with fundus above umbilicus
- Extremities: Superficial abrasions to bilateral upper extremities, no deformities noted
- Neuro: Unresponsive, Glasgow Coma Scale of 3
- Skin: Pale, cool, dry, multiple superficial abrasions to bilateral upper extremities

Learning Points

Background

During late pregnancy, the body goes through several physiologic changes including increase in blood volume and cardiac output by 30–40% above the nonpregnant state. Systemic shock becomes clinically apparent once the mother has lost more than 40% of her blood volume, whereas in a nonpregnant patient, signs of shock may start to manifest after a 15% blood loss. Additionally, an enlarged uterus can cause hypotension in late pregnancy because of space-occupying compression of the inferior vena cava (IVC) as well as elevation of the diaphragm by 4 cm, on average, resulting in a 20% decrease in functional residual lung capacity [1].

Maternal cardiac arrests occur with an incidence of about 1 in 30,000 pregnancies. Therefore, most emergency medicine physicians will never encounter such a situation [2]. However, trauma is also the leading cause of death in women of reproductive age and accounts for 25–50% of maternal morbidity [2]. There is a 45–50% fetal loss rate associated with major maternal injury [3].

The primary goal of peri/post-mortem cesarean section (PMCS) delivery is to increase the chance of successfully reviving a gravid mother (greater than 20 weeks of gestation) in the event of cardiopulmonary arrest lasting longer than 4 minutes despite effective CPR. Improved fetal neurologic outcomes and increased chances of maternal return of spontaneous circulation (ROSC) have been linked to the delivery of the fetus within 4 minutes of cardiac arrest [4]. However, a case series review discovered that the average time from arrest to birth due to PMCS was 16 minutes; only 7% of cases initiated PMCS within 4 minutes [5]. Approximately 90% of PMCS also took more than 1 minute to perform [4]. In 31.7% of cases, PMCS was deemed advantageous for the mother [5, 6].

Differential Diagnosis The most common causes of maternal arrest include cardiac disease, hemorrhage, amniotic fluid embolism, thromboembolism, sepsis, peripartum cardiomyopathy, preeclampsia/eclampsia, and trauma. The leading cause of death among pregnant patients is cardiac disease, most commonly from myocardial infarction [2, 4, 7].

History and Physical Exam

When presented with cardiac arrest in a pregnant patient, determine the time of the loss of pulses. This will be the first step in determining if a PMCS should be performed. Ideally, the decision to perform a PMCS is made within the first 4 minutes of resuscitation for cardiac arrest, utilizing the next minute for the procedure. Determine if there could be any reversible causes of maternal cardiac arrests occurring (i.e., differential diagnosis) by obtaining a brief history of the context of the cardiac arrest and the patient's medical and pregnancy history to help guide the resuscitation. It is important to keep in mind that the common clinical signs of shock such as hypotension and tachycardia do not manifest till the patient has experienced 40% or more of blood volume loss [1]. Lastly, palpate the patient's abdomen to determine if the uterine fundus is at or above the umbilicus. This crude measurement will generally correlate with a fetal age of 20 weeks' gestation or more [8] (Fig. 11.1). This is another key aspect to determine whether the patient is a good candidate for PMCS as the procedure should not be performed if the fetus is not of viable age [2]. If the last menstrual period or fetal age confirmed by ultrasound is available, it will similarly be helpful for decision-making.

Management

The primary focus of managing a pregnant patient in cardiac arrest is on optimal resuscitation of the mother. The best fetal outcomes will first rely on the appropriate perfusion of the mother. Overall, the management of the pregnant patient in cardiac arrest follows the same algorithms as the nonpregnant patient, with a few special considerations.

Efforts for resuscitation should initially follow either advanced cardiovascular life support or advanced trauma life support algorithms by which the team should

Fig. 11.1 Fetal age estimation by fundus height

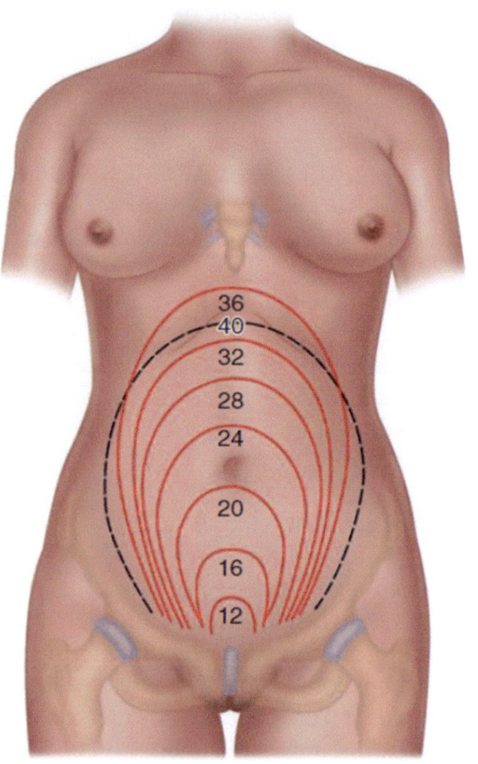

navigate the patient's airway, breathing, and circulation using chest compressions, airway management, augmented ventilation, medications, and electrotherapy as indicated. Chest compressions may need to be performed 2–3 cm higher on the sternum of a gravid patient with a large fundus to be most effective in squeezing the higher riding heart while being less injurious to the fetus [7].

Airway

Standard airway maneuvers should be performed including head tilt, chin tilt, and jaw thrust as indicated. Preparation for advance airway management should be anticipated with the most experienced physician undertaking the intubation [3]. During the third trimester, there is a physiologic narrowing of the airway, so it is recommended to consider using a slightly smaller endotracheal tube than typical for the patient's size. Other items which may facilitate the intubation procedure include a gum bougie, short laryngoscope handle, and backup stylets readily available [3]. Medications used for rapid sequence intubation (RSI) are as per the remainder of the population. RSI is preferred if the patient is *in extremis* but has not yet lost pulses to decrease risk of aspiration from the pressure of the uterus on the stomach and relative laxity of the gastric sphincter [1, 7].

Breathing

Pregnancy leads to higher levels of oxygen consumption and demand, leading to faster deoxygenation during cardiac arrest. The patient should be started on supplemental oxygen flow of 10–15 L/min by face mask or by endotracheal tube regardless of saturation, with a goal oxygen saturation of 94–98% [7]. There might be concern raised for high oxygen supplementation potentially being detrimental to the fetus *in utero*. Certainly, oxygen administration may increase the need for neonatal resuscitation; however, the mother's ventilation and perfusion must be prioritized in the case of a critically ill mother in cardiac arrest [7].

Circulation

Large bore peripheral intravenous catheters, ideally positioned above the diaphragm due to uterine compression of the IVC, facilitate aggressive volume resuscitation, irrespective of blood pressure measurement. Hypervolemia and hemodilution in pregnancy can mask underlying blood loss [3]. As with any trauma patient, blood products should be ordered and administered early as indicated. Additionally, an easily overlooked aspect of circulatory resuscitation in this population is to displace the gravid uterus from obstructing the IVC to improve cardiac output (Fig. 11.2). Manual uterine displacement to the left side of the patient is preferred as traditional tilting of the backboard to a 30-degree angle to the left may be difficult with ongoing chest compressions [7]. The uterus should be displaced with the "up, off and over" technique while the patient is in a supine position. This technique is performed by cupping the uterus with your hand from the right lateral side and lifting it up and left of the patient. Left lateral tilt of the patient can also be achieved using a solid wedge, stacked pillows, or folded blankets that extend from the patient's posterior shoulder to the pelvis [7].

Perimortem Cesarean Section

PMCS was introduced in 1986 to describe a cesarean section delivery performed when ROSC has not occurred within the first four minutes of cardiopulmonary resuscitation [2]. It is a means of relieving the circulatory stress on the mother in the case of cardiopulmonary failure. The procedure is best performed by a qualified surgeon in the operating room; however, circumstances typically necessitate the procedure is performed in the ED. The procedure is within the scope of a qualified emergency physician's skillset, should it be necessary.

Primary Goals [9]

- Optimize maternal resuscitation primarily

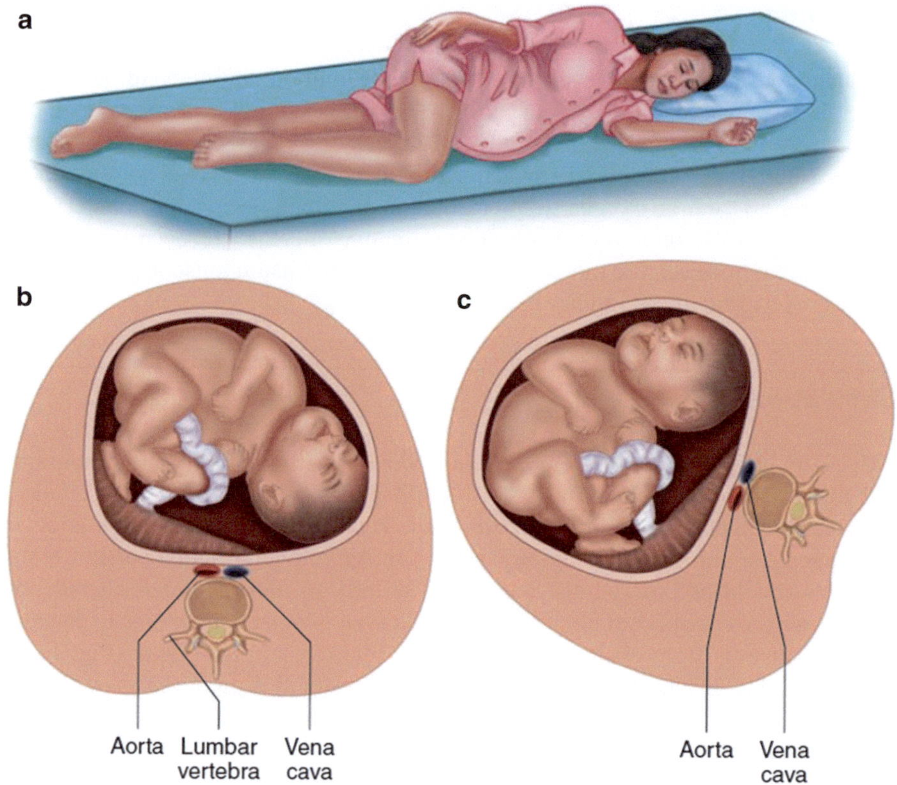

Fig 11.2 (**a**) Left lateral decubitus positioning of a resting patient. (**b**) Fetus compressing the great vessels of the abdomen with mother supine. (**c**) Release great vessel compression with manual uterine displacement

- Reduce physical obstruction/compression of IVC and aorta to increase preload
- Improve respiratory mechanics: optimal lung volumes, compliance, and diaphragm movement
- Reduce maternal oxygen demand by eliminating the significant fetus and placental shunt

Indications The PMCS procedure should be performed in a patient in cardiac arrest who is greater than 20 weeks of gestation (fundus is palpated above the umbilicus) for whom ROSC has not been achieved within 4 minutes of the arrest [8]. Traditionally, PMCS is taught to be performed at 24 weeks, as fetal survival rate for those above 24 weeks is around 71.6% [10]. However, clinically in the emergency department, while actively resuscitating a quite ill gravid patient, accurate fetal dates may not be readily available. Nonetheless, the primary goal of PMCS is to resuscitate the mother not the fetus.

The current approach for PMCS is to adhere to the four minutes of cardiopulmonary resuscitative efforts with an attempt to deliver the fetus within the next minute. Though this is the approach, there is no evidence that four minutes confirms a survival threshold. However, Benson et al. found in 2016 that maternal and fetal mortality rates steadily and predictably decline from the time of cardiac arrest to the time of birth. Realistically, from skin incision to delivery in one minute or less occurred in less than 10% of women experiencing PMCS [6]. Once a decision has been made that the patient is a good candidate for PMCS and the decision is made to deliver the fetus, a physician should proceed with the cesarean section as soon as possible [6].

Contraindications A PMCS should not be imminently pursued if there is a suspected serious brain injury in a hemodynamically stable patient, especially if the fetus is not in distress.

If the clinical picture does not suggest that an infant would be able to be appropriately resuscitated after delivery, PMCS should not be performed. This scenario is most encountered in extreme cases of prematurity (i.e., less than 20 weeks gestational age) [2].

Equipment Thoracotomy tray, scalpel (#10 blade), Mayo scissors, and 2 Kelly clamps.

Due to the time-sensitive nature of PMCS, neither consent, general preoperative preparation, full operative sterile technique, analgesia, nor transport to the operating room is required or recommended.

Those interacting with the patient should wear personal protective equipment.

Procedure [1, 2] The patient should continue to receive advanced cardiopulmonary resuscitation.

1. Using a scalpel, make a vertical cutaneous incision from the xyphoid extending to about 2–3 cm above the pubic symphysis
2. Cut through subcutaneous tissue, stopping at the peritoneal wall
3. Using blunt dissection, open the peritoneum using fingers and traction
4. Cut the peritoneum vertically starting inferiorly with scissors (may be easier) or scalpel
5. Deliver the uterus
6. Make a vertical incision extending toward the chest at the lower half of the uterine body, avoiding the placenta, bowel, and bladder until the baby is exposed
7. Deliver the baby, placing 2 clamps on the cord and cut in between the clamps
8. Hand the baby off for evaluation and resuscitation
9. Deliver the placenta

10. Place packing/towels in the opened uterus and abdomen until exploration and closure can occur in the operating room

Once the uterus and abdomen have been packed, the incision can be temporarily closed with towel clamps or can be left open. Cardiopulmonary resuscitation should continue throughout PMCS and after the completion of the procedure until ROSC is achieved or there is a decision to cease resuscitative efforts. If ROSC is achieved, intravenous antibiotics, vasopressors, inotropes, and blood products can be given expeditiously. Though there might be some hemorrhage from the operative site, oxytocin or other uterotonic agents could potentially precipitate cardiac arrest, so caution is recommended regarding their use [4].

Consultation Considerations

Participation of an interprofessional team can increase the likelihood of a successful PMCS. Though the procedure can be performed by an obstetrician, a general surgeon, or an emergency physician, the person *present* with the most surgical experience ideally should be the one to perform this high-stakes procedure.

It is of utmost importance to consult an obstetrician as soon as a PMCS is considered. The obstetrician will likely be responsible for the continued resuscitation and operative closure of uterus and peritoneum if ROSC is obtained. The obstetrician, likely with the resources and personnel of a critical care setting, will ultimately manage the patient post-arrest and the post-operative course.

Any available surgeon proficient with intraabdominal surgical procedures (e.g., general surgeon, trauma surgeon) could potentially be helpful with the surgical maneuvers involved in a PMCS if an obstetrician is not available.

A pediatric specialist, particularly a neonatologist should also be notified as soon as PMCS is considered. The priority in a PMCS is the resuscitation of the mother, however, once the fetus has been delivered, rapid assessment and targeted medical intervention would be necessary to facilitate the best outcomes for the baby as well.

Emergency Department Course and Outcome

The emergency team commenced cardiorespiratory resuscitation along with massive transfusion with the trauma surgeon at bedside. They manually displaced the uterus to the left decubitus position of the patient to relieve compression of the IVC. Two large bore IVs were inserted above the diaphragm, and another isotonic fluid bolus was administered. Despite optimal resuscitative efforts, there was no spontaneous return of circulation after four minutes of quality CPR. The team decided that a perimortem cesarean section would be an appropriate intervention for maternal resuscitation.

The obstetrician was paged but they were unfortunately preoccupied completing a case in the operating room (OR) and would work with the OR team to prepare a room upon transfer of care of this patient. The neonatologist was paged and arrived in the ED with an intensive care nurse and an infant warmer.

As resuscitation continued, PMCS was performed and within the next 3 minutes the baby was delivered, the umbilicus was clamped and cut, and the baby's care was transitioned to the neonatology team. The patient's uterus and abdomen were packed tightly with gauze. A thready pulse was identified at the next timed interval for a pulse check. The obstetrician arrived in the ED to evaluate the patient and the situation. With the OR and obstetrician now prepared, patient care was transferred to the obstetrician and trauma surgeon for continued workup and management.

Key Points

- The primary aim of the perimortem cesarean section is to prioritize increasing the chances of successfully reviving the mother of a fetus greater than 20 weeks gestational age.
- Ideally, a perimortem cesarean section should be performed within the fifth minute after 4 minutes of failure to achieve return of spontaneous circulation, though practically this time-mark is rare.
- The maternal benefits of a perimortem cesarean section include relief of compression of the great vessels of the abdomen, improved pulmonary mechanics, and reduced oxygen demand.
- The optimal surgical approach for a perimortem cesarean section is a large vertical incision from the xyphoid to the pubic symphysis through the uterus while attempting to avoid damage to other structures.

References

1. Boyd A. CORE EM: Peri-Mortem C-Section. emDocs. 2016. http://www.emdocs.net/core-em-peri-mortem-c-section. Accessed 2 Jan 2023.
2. Linares S. Perimortem Cesarean Section. In: Reichman EF, editor. Emergency medicine procedures, 2e. McGraw Hill. 2013. https://accessemergencymedicine.mhmedical.com/Content.aspx?bookid=683§ionid=45343781. Accessed 27 Jan 2023.
3. Burns BD, Fisher ES. Resuscitation in Pregnancy. In: Tintinalli JE, Ma O, Yealy DM, Meckler GD, Stapczynski J, Cline DM, Thomas SH, editor. Tintinalli's emergency medicine: a comprehensive study guide, 9e. McGraw Hill. 2020. https://accessmedicine-mhmedical-com.proxy-hs.researchport.umd.edu/content.aspx?bookid=2353§ionid=206322334. Accessed 27 Jan 2023.
4. Healy ME, Kozubal DE, Horn AE, Vilke GM, Chan TC, Ufberg JW. Care of the critically ill pregnant patient and perimortem cesarean delivery in the emergency department. J Emerg Med. 2016;51(2):172–7. https://doi.org/10.1016/j.jemermed.2016.04.029.
5. Einav S, Kaufman N, Sela HY. Maternal cardiac arrest and perimortem caesarean delivery: Evidence or expert-based? Resuscitation. 2012;83(10):1191–200. https://doi.org/10.1016/j.resuscitation.2012.05.005.
6. Benson MD, Padovano A, Bourjeily G, Zhou Y. Maternal collapse: challenging the four-minute rule. EBioMedicine. 2016;6:253–7. https://doi.org/10.1016/j.ebiom.2016.02.042.

7. Chu JJ, Hinshaw K, Paterson-Brown S, Johnston T, Matthews M, Webb J, Sharpe P. Perimortem caesarean section – why, when and how. Obstet Gynecol. 2018;20:151–8. https://doi.org/10.1111/tog.12493.
8. Smith KA, Bryce S. Trauma in the pregnant patient: an evidence-based approach to management. Emerg Med Pract. 2013;15(4):1–18. Update in: Emerg Med Pract. 2020 Oct 15;22(Suppl 10):1–36.
9. Faust J, Westafer L. Episode 60 – Resuscitative Hysterotomy + First Trimester Emergencies. FOAMcast—An Emergency Medicine Podcast. 2016. https://foamcast.org/2016/11/25/episode-60-resuscitative-hysterotomy-first-trimester-emergencies/. Accessed 26 Jan 2023.
10. Qattea I, Farghaly MAA, Kattea MO, Abdula N, Mohamed MA, Aly H. Survival of infants born at periviable gestation: The US national database. Lancet Reg Health Am. 2022;25(14):100330. https://doi.org/10.1016/j.lana.2022.100330.

Shoulder Dystocia

Stuck in the Middle with You

Carolina Camacho Ruiz

Case

A 36-year-old patient, G5P4 assigned female at birth presented to a community emergency department in active labor. Emergency medical services reported "her water broke" soon after picking up the patient. While in her bed in the emergency department (ED), the patient emphatically explains that she has been having contractions. She has been pushing and feels like she has to keep pushing!

- Past medical history: Fifth pregnancy (G5P4), normal prenatal course to date.
- Past surgical history: None
- Medications: Prenatal vitamins
- Allergies: No known drug allergies
- Family history: Mother has diabetes
- Social history: Non-smoker, no alcohol, no illicit drug use

Physical Exam

- Vital signs
  - Heart rate: 110 beats/minute
  - Blood pressure: 130/70 mmHg
  - Respiratory rate: 24 breaths/minute
  - Temperature: 98.2 °F
  - Oxygen saturation: 98% on room air

C. Camacho Ruiz (✉)
Department of Emergency Medicine, State University of New York Downstate Health Sciences University/King's County Hospital, Brooklyn, NY, USA

A. A. Kosoko (ed.), *Emergency Medicine Case-Based Guide*,
https://doi.org/10.1007/978-3-031-70118-4_12

- General appearance: Appears stated age, in distress
- Heart: Tachycardia, regular rhythm, equal pulses
- Lungs: Tachypneic, Lamaze breathing, speaking in complete sentences, clear on auscultation
- Abdominal/GI: Soft, non-tender bowel sounds present, gravid with fundus above the umbilicus
- Genitourinary: Fetal head crowning; despite pushing with contractions, the fetal head retracts toward the perineum; no nuchal cord detected
- Rectal: Normal
- Extremities: No pitting edema, no tenderness, no deformity, tolerates a full range of motion
- Back: Normal
- Neuro: Alert, oriented, utilizing four extremities
- Skin: Normal
- Psych: Normal

Learning Points

Background

Shoulder dystocia (SD) is a rare complication of vaginal births when the fetal shoulders prevent progression of labor due to impaction of the shoulders at the pelvic outlet [1]. Most commonly, the anterior shoulder impacts on the maternal pubic symphysis. More specifically, SD is defined as a delivery that requires additional obstetric maneuvers to deliver the shoulders after expectant gentle downward traction on the fetal head alone is unsuccessful in facilitating delivery [2]. According to Ouzounian [2], SD complicates about 1% of vaginal deliveries. It is a true obstetric emergency and an unpredictable and unpreventable event. Nonetheless, risk factors which increase the probability of SD include a mother with diabetes mellitus, obesity, multiparity, post-term gestation, and previous history of SD. The most important fetal risk factor is macrosomia (often related to maternal gestational diabetes mellitus). However, multiple studies have shown that predicting SD is difficult, even when risk factors are present. Most SD cases occur even without major risk factors [3, 4].

Maternal complications of SD include a higher rate of postpartum hemorrhage and complicated vaginal lacerations (Table 12.1) [5]. Major neonatal complications due to SD include brachial plexus palsies, fractures of the clavicle and humerus, hypoxic-ischemic encephalopathy, and neonatal death (Table 12.1) [6].

Differential Diagnosis Umbilical cord prolapse, breech delivery, physiologic emergent delivery, fetal macrosomia, fetal malformation, conjoined twins.

Table 12.1 Major sequelae of shoulder dystocia

Carrier complications	Fetus/newborn complications
Uterine rupture	Brachial plexopathies
Postpartum hemorrhage	Facial nerve paralysis
Tissue damage to the cervix, vagina, bladder, urethra, anal sphincter, or rectum	Horner syndrome
Symphyseal separation	Clavicular fracture
	Humerus fracture
	Permanent brachial plexus injury
	Hypoxic-ischemic encephalopathy
	Death

History and Physical Exam

Patients will present to the emergency department in active precipitous labor. As time allows, the prenatal history and maternal health history should be obtained to risk stratify for SD: maternal diabetes, number of and general course of any previous pregnancies and deliveries, gestational age, and any prenatal complications.

The physical exam should first obtain vital signs and a brief general evaluation of the cardiovascular and respiratory status of the patient. Abdominal and genitourinary evaluation is then key to determining whether labor is progressing normally or if SD is occurring. The exam will focus on the perineum.

Turtle sign occurs when the fetal head is visible at the perineum but retracts after contractions instead of advancing past the perineum [2]. Other signs of SD include difficulty with delivery of the face and chin of the fetus, failure of restitution of the fetal head, and/or failure of the shoulders to descend [5]. A concerning but contested finding on physical exam is the time for delivery of the head to the time for delivery of the body of the fetus taking more than 1 minute [7]. According to most recent practice guidelines, the American College of Obstetricians and Gynecologists does not currently accept this as a reliable finding suggestive of SD. Lastly, if the delivery requires any additional obstetric maneuvers after unsuccessful simple gentle traction on the fetal head in delivery of the shoulders, SD is to be suspected.

Laboratory Studies

Shoulder dystocia is a clinical diagnosis. Laboratory studies will not aid diagnosis.

Imaging Findings

Shoulder dystocia is a clinical diagnosis. Imaging findings will not aid diagnosis.

Management

Shoulder dystocia requires rapid diagnosis and timely interventions for optimal outcomes. The first step is a call for help from obstetrics services for fetal monitoring and anticipating escalation of care. In the event of unsuccessful bedside maneuvers, a *stat* cesarean section delivery may be necessary. The rapid implementation of bedside maneuvers correlates to a reduction in the duration of the shoulder dystocia and will decrease rates and severity of neonatal hypoxic-ischemic injury [7].

First-line maneuvers are selected for being less invasive and requiring less manipulation of the fetus.

McRoberts Maneuver and Suprapubic Pressure

The McRoberts maneuver (Fig. 12.1) requires hyperflexion (abduction) of the patient's legs at the hips at a sharp angle to the abdomen. The patient can assume this position with the active manual assistance of others. This movement causes a cephalad rotation of the symphysis pubis and flattening of the lumbar lordosis associated with pregnancy, mechanically relieving the impacted shoulder [8].

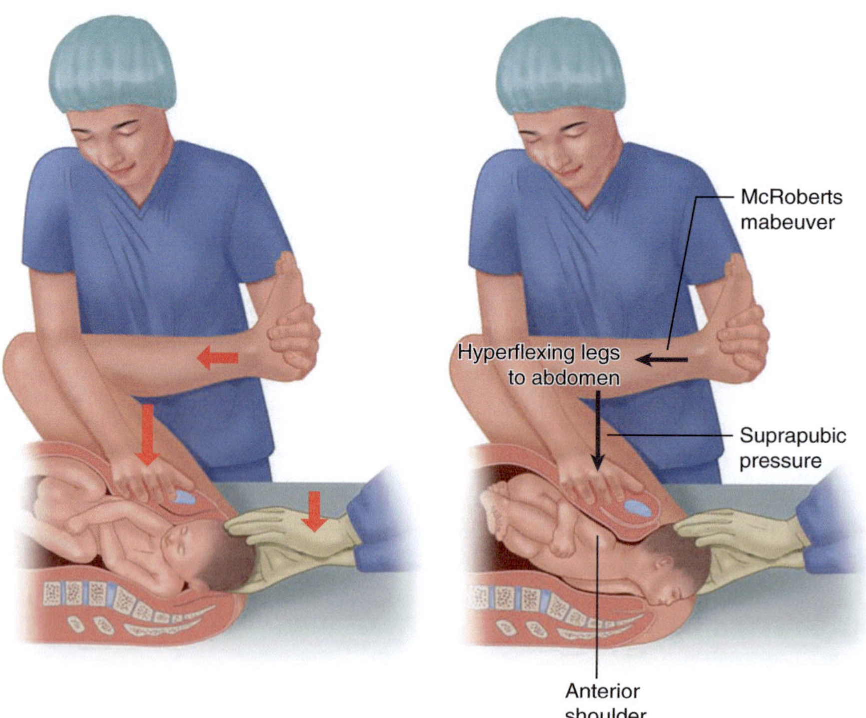

Fig. 12.1 McRoberts maneuver

The McRoberts maneuver is performed combined with suprapubic pressure to optimize advancement of the fetus with coordinated pushing. A person applies continuous emphatic pressure at the suprapubic region at an oblique angle above the symphysis pubis using the palms of the hands. This decreases the distance between the outermost points of the fetal shoulders and rotates the anterior fetal shoulder into the wider oblique pelvic diameter [8].

These two maneuvers together simultaneously help to move the shoulder underneath the symphysis pubis. Gentle routine traction in the axial direction of the fetal head can be used to assess if the prior steps released the impacted shoulder.

The McRoberts maneuver with suprapubic pressure has the lowest risk of neonatal injury compared to other interventions available bedside for SD [6]. Hoffman et al. [6] reported that the McRoberts maneuver with suprapubic pressure technique is effective in relieving 24% of shoulder dystocia cases.

Second-line maneuvers are selected for being more invasive for the mother and fetus and require more manipulation of the fetus.

Posterior Arm and Shoulder Delivery

During labor in general, the posterior fetal arm is usually held flexed. If the first-line techniques fail, a physician can reach into the introitus to attempt to relieve the SD. Once grasped between fingers, the arm can be swept across the fetal chest and gently withdrawn and straightened outside the perineum (Fig. 12.2) [9]. If the delivery of the posterior shoulder and arm is successful, the anterior shoulder typically follows in delivery.

Delivering the posterior arm and shoulder to relieve SD risks neonatal humeral fracture. Fortunately, neonatal humerus fractures generally heal without significant

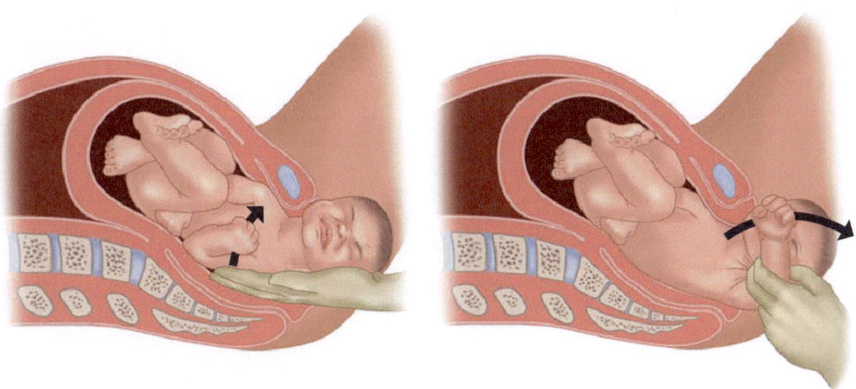

Fig. 12.2 Delivery of the posterior shoulder

complications [8]. Hoffman et al. [6] found that delivery of the posterior arm and shoulder was the most effective maneuver (84%) to acutely relieve SD at the bedside, and rates of injury are low (8%).

Woods' Corkscrew Maneuver and Rubin's Maneuver

These two maneuvers utilize rotational forces applied to assist the fetus to descend.

The Woods' corkscrew maneuver is the preferred method when the anterior surface of the posterior shoulder is most accessible. The provider places a hand on the anterior aspect of the posterior fetal shoulder and rotates the shoulder 180 degrees in a corkscrew fashion (clockwise) to release the opposite impacted shoulder (Fig. 12.3). Hoffman et al. [6] found Woods' corkscrew maneuver to have a success rate of 72%, with an associated neonatal injury (brachial plexus injury, clavicle or humeral fracture, hypoxic brain injury, or rarely death) rate of 9.5%.

Rubin's II maneuver is another rotational movement that can be performed if the anterior shoulder is more accessible than the posterior one. Rubin's II maneuver requires placing the provider's hand on the posterior aspect of the anterior shoulder

Fig. 12.3 Woods' corkscrew maneuver

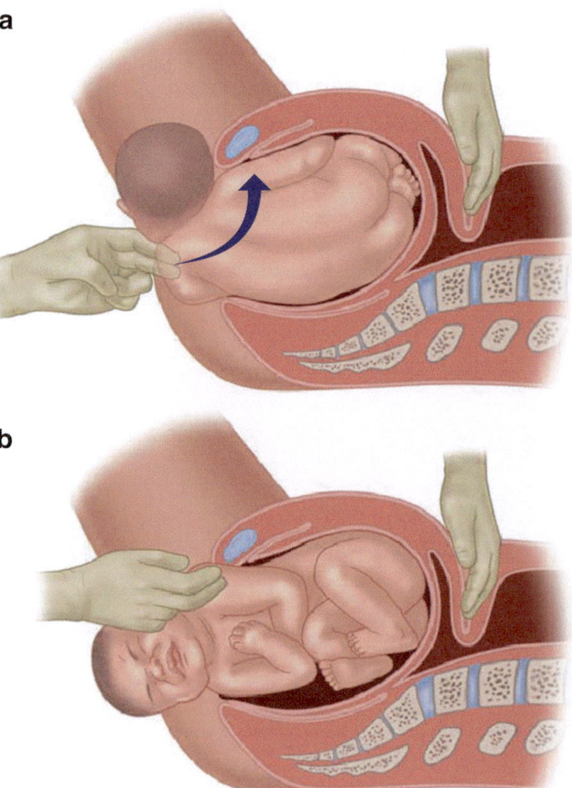

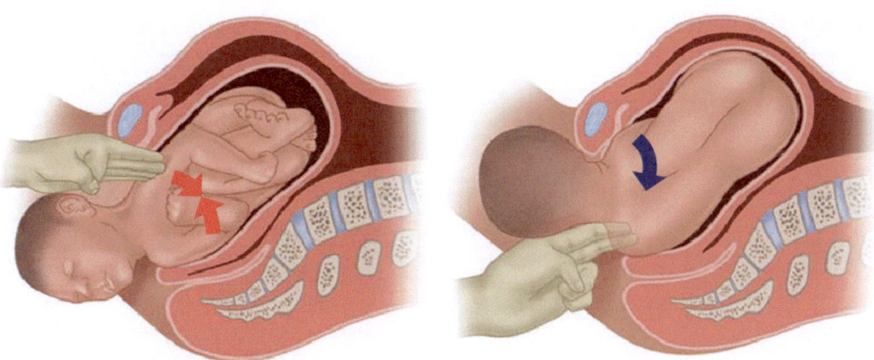

Fig. 12.4 Rubin's II maneuver

and rotating toward the fetal chest about 30 degrees (Fig. 12.4) [9]. This movement allows the anterior shoulder to turn away from the symphysis pubis. Hoffman et al. [6] found Rubin's II maneuver slightly less effective and riskier than Woods' corkscrew maneuver, achieving resolution in 66% of cases and having a 14% injury rate. It is important to note that the lower success rates and the higher injury rates may be intrinsically due to the cases being more complex, already requiring secondary maneuvers to relieve SD.

Woods' corkscrew maneuver and Rubin's II maneuver can be combined by placing one hand on the front side of the posterior shoulder and the other on the back of the anterior shoulder, allowing a fetal rotation of 180 degrees [9, 10]. However, combining these techniques may require an episiotomy to allow access for both hands of the provider to facilitate the birth.

Gaskin Maneuver

The Gaskin maneuver is an option when a patient can stand and walk during the labor process (Fig. 12.5). Assist the patient to an "all-fours" position, wherein the body weight is balanced on the hands and knees. Then, apply gentle downward traction to the posterior shoulder or upward traction to the anterior shoulder [9–12].

According to Dahlke et al. [8], effective implementation of these first- and second-line maneuvers will resolve 99% of all shoulder dystocia cases. Sometimes, a case will require performing a maneuver more than once in preparation for the third-line options. At this point, the care team should be preparing for more invasive measurements, including up to a cesarean section.

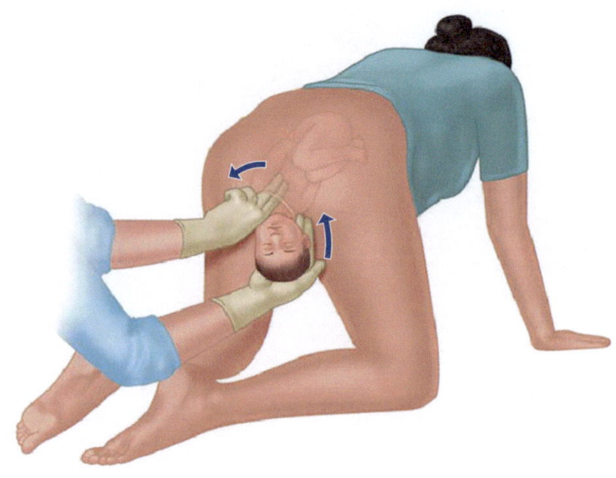

Fig. 12.5 Gaskin maneuver

Last Resort Maneuvers

Zavanelli Maneuver

The Zavanelli maneuver can be considered if other tactics have failed. In this technique, the fetal head is turned in the occiput anterior position, flexed from the extended position, then pushed back into the pelvis [9, 10]. When performing this maneuver, tocolytics are often administered to produce uterine relaxation. *A cesarian section needs to be performed immediately after completing this maneuver.* The procedure should never be considered if the umbilical cord was manipulated during the labor.

The Zavanelli maneuver is uncommon (0.001% of all deliveries) [8]. The maternal risk is unknown, but the procedure is associated with neonatal hypoxic-ischemic injury and brachial plexus palsies [8].

Clavicle Fracture

The fetal clavicle is intentionally fractured by pulling the anterior clavicle outward at the middle portion of the bone. The fetal clavicle is a strong bone, but if it is intentionally fractured, it can decrease the biacromial diameter, facilitating delivery when navigating SD [12]. This procedure can be physically challenging to execute and may injure the fetus's vascular or lung structures.

Episiotomy

The performance of an episiotomy is not a mandatory step in the management of shoulder dystocia, as recommended by the American College of Obstetricians and Gynecologists. The systematic review of 14 articles by Sagi-Dain and Sagi [13] found no evidence for the benefits of episiotomy performance in the prevention and management of shoulder dystocia. Routine episiotomy during shoulder dystocia delivery can be unnecessary but should be considered if additional room is needed in the posterior vagina to rotate the fetus or extract an arm [12].

Symphysiotomy
This technique is the last resort and can be performed at the bedside when a cesarian section is not readily available, other methods to relieve SD have failed, and there are no other safe alternative options. Symphysiotomy is a surgical division of the pubic symphysis under local anesthesia. The skin, subcutaneous tissue, and anterior fibers of the pubic symphysis are incised with a scalpel to increase the pelvic diameter [10, 11]. The procedure has high risks of urinary system injury, fistulas, and chronic difficulties with pain and gait for the mother.

Consultation Considerations

The obstetrics team should be consulted as soon as there is a concern for SD. An obstetrician can be helpful in performing bedside maneuvers to release SD, and ultimately deliver the baby in the operating room by cesarean section if bedside maneuvers are unsuccessful, in order to achieve the best outcomes for the mother and the child. Furthermore, the obstetrician would need to manage any maternal complications sustained from bedside maneuvers attempted to relieve SD.

Similarly, as soon as SD is suspected, as with any precipitous birth, a neonatal team should be consulted to help evaluate the newborn for any complications from the delivery and resuscitate if needed.

Emergency Department Course and Outcome

The emergency team recognized a precipitous birth occurring but not progressing, despite coordinated breathing and pushing performed by the patient. The emergency physician suspected shoulder dystocia and immediately had the obstetric team and neonatal team notified of the complicated delivery. The anesthesia team began to prepare the operating room for a possible cesarean section.

The emergency physician attempted the McRoberts maneuver and suprapubic pressure with the help of the emergency department nurses. After two more pushes and what looked like turtle sign, the emergency physician grasped the posterior fetal arm, swept it across the chest, and withdrew it in a straight line. The mother gave another coordinated push which led to delivery of the anterior shoulder then the rest of the fetal body without complications.

The neonatal resuscitation team examined the baby, who was large for gestational age but was breathing normally and had a normal blood glucose. There was no sign of a humerus fracture. The obstetrics team took over care of the mother for repair of an incidental vaginal laceration and for delivery of the placenta. Both mother and baby were admitted for observation without further complications during their hospital course.

Key Points

As a risk management approach, Posner et al., in the book *Human Labor and Birth*, suggest the mnemonic "ALARMER" as a stepwise approach for managing shoulder dystocia which is applicable in the emergency setting (Fig. 12.6).

A—Ask for help
L—Lift legs (McRoberts)
A—Anterior shoulder delivery (suprapubic pressure)
R—Rotate (Woods' corkscrew maneuver)
M—Manual removal of the posterior arm and shoulder
E—Evaluate for episiotomy
R—Repeat the listed steps

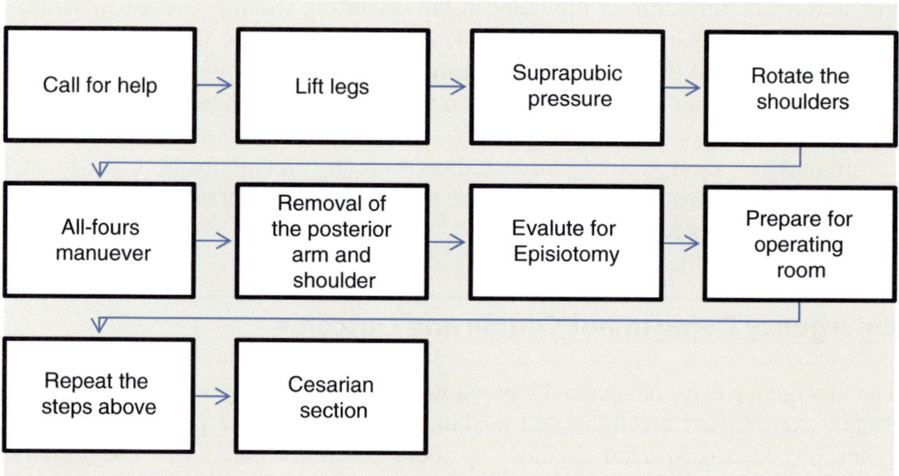

Fig. 12.6 Algorithm for shoulder dystocia management

References

1. Sarah EF, Kathleen K. Emergency delivery. In: Tintinalli JE, Ma OJ, Yealy DM, Meckler GD, Stapczynski JS, Cline DM, Thomas SH, editors. Tintinalli's emergency medicine: a comprehensive study guide, 9e. New York: McGraw-Hill Education; 2020.
2. Ouzounian JG. Shoulder dystocia: incidence and risk factors. Clin Obstet Gynecol. 2016;59(4):791–4. https://doi.org/10.1097/GRF.0000000000000227.
3. Practice Bulletin No 178: shoulder dystocia. Obstet Gynecol. 2017;129(5):e123–33. https://doi.org/10.1097/AOG.0000000000002043.
4. Mehta SH, Sokol RJ. Shoulder dystocia: risk factors, predictability, and preventability. Semin Perinatol. 2014;38(4):189–93. https://doi.org/10.1053/j.semperi.2014.04.003.
5. Hansen A, Chauhan SP. Shoulder dystocia: definitions and incidence. Semin Perinatol. 2014;38(4):184–8. https://doi.org/10.1053/j.semperi.2014.04.002.
6. Hoffman MK, Bailit JL, Branch DW, Burkman RT, Van Veldhusien P, Lu L, et al. A comparison of obstetric maneuvers for the acute management of shoulder dystocia. Obstet Gynecol. 2011;117(6):1272–8. https://doi.org/10.1097/AOG.0b013e31821a12c9.
7. Chauhan SP, Gherman RB. Shoulder dystocia: challenging basic assumptions. Obstet Gynecol Clin N Am. 2022;49(3):491–500. https://doi.org/10.1016/j.ogc.2022.02.005.
8. Dahlke JD, Bhalwal A, Chauhan SP. Obstetric emergencies: shoulder dystocia and postpartum hemorrhage. Obstet Gynecol Clin N Am. 2017;44(2):231–43. https://doi.org/10.1016/j.ogc.2017.02.003.
9. Hill DA, Lense J, Roepcke F. Shoulder dystocia: managing an obstetric emergency. Am Fam Physician. 2020;102(2):84–90.
10. Bothou A, Apostolidi DM, Tsikouras P, Iatrakis G, Sarella A, Iatrakis D, et al. Overview of techniques to manage shoulder dystocia during vaginal birth. Eur J Midwifery. 2021;5:48. https://doi.org/10.18332/ejm/142097.
11. Gilstrop M, Hoffman MK. An update on the acute management of shoulder dystocia. Clin Obstet Gynecol. 2016;59(4):813–9. https://doi.org/10.1097/GRF.0000000000000240.
12. Chauhan SP, Gherman R, Hendrix NW, Bingham JM, Hayes E. Shoulder dystocia: comparison of the ACOG practice bulletin with another national guideline. Am J Perinatol. 2010;27(2):129–36. https://doi.org/10.1055/s-0029-1224864.
13. Sagi-Dain L, Sagi S. The role of episiotomy in prevention and management of shoulder dystocia: a systematic review. Obstet Gynecol Surv. 2015;70(5):354–62. https://doi.org/10.1097/OGX.0000000000000179.

The Bleeding Won't Stop

Peter Acker

Case

A 39-year-old woman, G5P5, presents via emergency medical services (EMS) after a midwife-assisted home delivery at 38 weeks for evaluation of heavy vaginal bleeding. The patient's pregnancy had been generally unremarkable. She experienced labor for 6 hours prior to vaginally delivering a healthy appearing neonate approximately 3 hours prior to arrival to the emergency department (ED). After delivery, she experienced persistent, moderate-volume vaginal bleeding. An hour prior to arrival at the ED, the amount of bleeding increased, and the patient began feeling fatigued and lightheaded. Upon noting the change in symptoms, the midwife called EMS for transport.

- Past medical history: Obesity, uterine fibroids
- Past surgical history: None
- Medications: Prenatal vitamins
- Allergies: No known drug allergies
- Family history: None
- Social history: Non-smoker, no alcohol, no illicit drug use

Physical Exam

- Vital signs
  - Heart rate: 122 beats/minute
  - Blood pressure: 102/85 mmHg
  - Respiratory rate: 24 breaths/minute

P. Acker (✉)
Department of Emergency Medicine, Stanford University School of Medicine, Stanford, CA, USA
e-mail: packer@stanford.edu

© The Author(s), under exclusive license to Springer Nature Switzerland AG 2024
A. A. Kosoko (ed.), *Emergency Medicine Case-Based Guide*,
https://doi.org/10.1007/978-3-031-70118-4_13

- – Temperature: 98 °F
- – Oxygen saturation: 97% on room air
- General appearance: Appears stated age, lying on gurney, slightly pale, appears fatigued
- HEENT
  - – Head: Atraumatic, normocephalic
  - – Eyes: Pupils equal, round, and reactive to light (4–2 mm), external ocular movements are normal, conjunctiva appear pale
  - – Throat: No erythema or edema of the oropharynx, mild pallor to the oral mucosa
  - – Neck: Trachea midline, no stridor, no jugular venous distention
- Heart/cardiovascular: Tachycardia, regular rhythm, pulses intact in bilateral upper and lower extremities, capillary refill 3 seconds
- Lungs: Mildly tachypneic, speaks in full sentences, lungs clear to auscultation bilaterally
- Abdominal: Soft, nontender, bowel sounds present, boggy uterus palpated
- Genitourinary: Normal external genitalia, no obvious external lacerations, slow trickle of active vaginal bleeding noted, internal exam without lacerations, active bleeding through dilated cervix noted, no cord or evidence of placenta noted
- Rectal: Normal
- Extremities: Hands and feet cool to touch, no tenderness, no deformity, tolerates full range of motion
- Back: Normal
- Neuro: Alert and oriented, no gross deficits identified
- Skin: Normal

Pertinent Diagnostic Tests (Fig. 13.1 and Tables 13.1, 13.2, 13.3, 13.4, 13.5 and 13.6)

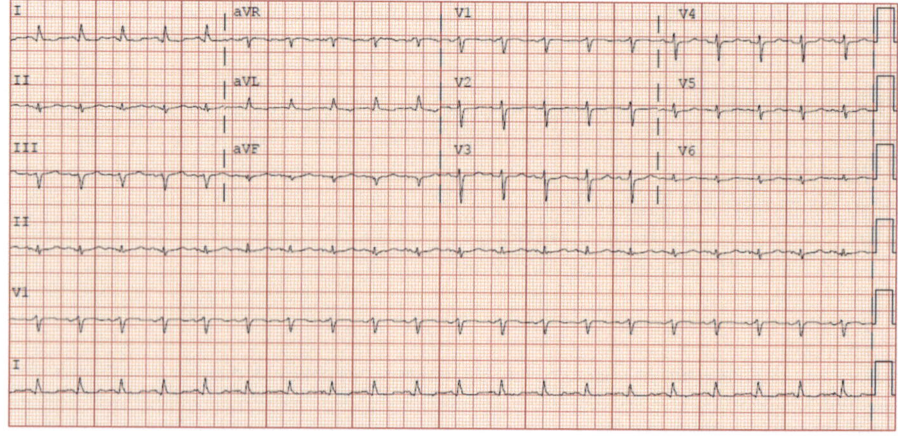

Fig. 13.1 Electrocardiogram (ECG): Sinus tachycardia. Left axis deviation. Non-specific lateral T-wave abnormalities. (Author's own image)

Table 13.1 Complete blood count

Complete blood count	
White blood cells	14×10^9/L
Hemoglobin	9.1 g/dL
Hematocrit	27%
Platelets	150×10^9/L

Table 13.2 Comprehensive metabolic panel

Comprehensive metabolic panel	
Sodium	140 mEq/L
Potassium	4.0 mEq/L
Chloride	110 mEq/L
Bicarbonate	26 mEq/L
Glucose	103 mg/dL
Blood urea nitrogen (BUN)	18 mg/dL
Creatinine	0.8 mg/dL
Calcium	8.8 mg/dL
Ionized calcium	1.21 mmol/L
Total bilirubin	0.6 mg/dL
Alkaline phosphatase	50 units/L
Aspartate aminotransferase (AST)	25 units/L
Alanine aminotransferase (ALT)	22 units/L
Albumin	3.5 g/dL
Total protein	6.7 g/dL

Table 13.3 Venous blood gas and lactic acid

Venous blood gas and lactic acid	
pH	7.29
pCO2	25 mmHg
pO2	50 mmHg
HCO3	12 mEq/L
Lactic acid	3.8 mEq/L

Table 13.4 Coagulopathy panel

Coagulopathy panel	
International normalized ratio (INR)	1.1
Prothrombin time (PT)	12.5 seconds
Activated partial thromboplastin time (aPTT)	29.3 seconds
D-Dimer	1400 ng/mL
Fibrinogen	303 mg/dL

Table 13.5 Blood type

Blood type	
ABO type	A
Rh(D) antigen	+

Table 13.6 Urinalysis

Urinalysis	
Color	Yellow
Appearance	Clear
Specific gravity	1.010
pH	7.0
Glucose	Negative
Bilirubin	Negative
Ketones	0
Protein	0
Leukocyte esterase	1+
Nitrites	Negative
White blood cells (WBCs)	1 WBC/high-power field (HPF)
Red blood cells (RBCs)	0 RBCs/HPF
Squamous epithelial cells	0–5 cells/HPF

Learning Points

Background

Postpartum hemorrhage (PPH) complicates 1–5% of all deliveries [1–3], accounting for 10% of all maternal deaths in the United States and 25% of all maternal deaths globally [1]. Unfortunately, there are stark racial disparities in maternal death rates in the United States. This is true for overall death rates as well as those directly attributable to PPH. Black women experience a greater than three-fold higher risk of death during pregnancy and the postpartum period, compared with white women [2].

In the past, a variety of criteria have been used to diagnose PPH, dependent on the means of birth and volume of blood loss. More recently, the American College of Obstetricians and Gynecologists (ACOG) updated their definition of PPH to:

> Blood loss of greater than 1,000 cc accompanied by signs or symptoms of hypovolemia regardless of the route of delivery [3].

However, this definition is generally impractical in an emergency setting. First, several studies have suggested that healthcare providers' ability to accurately quantify blood loss is limited [4–7]. Second, awaiting large volume blood loss prior to initiating corrective measures may delay essential care and worsen outcomes.

A more practical, actionable definition of PPH, particularly in the emergency setting is

> Vaginal blood loss after delivery (any route or timing) leading to hemodynamic instability and/or signs and/or symptoms of hypovolemia [8].

Overall, 5–6% of women who deliver in the United States seek care in the ED in the postpartum period, with approximately 0.5–3% of all deliveries seeking attention in the ED for postpartum bleeding [9]. Postpartum hemorrhage can occur at any

Table 13.7 Postpartum hemorrhage risk factors [11]

Postpartum hemorrhage risk factors
Asian, Hispanic, or African/African American descent [12]
Augmented labor
Chorioamnionitis
Episiotomy
History of postpartum hemorrhage
Operative delivery
Overdistended uterus (macrosomia, multiple gestations, hydramnios)
Preeclampsia
Prior uterine surgery
Prolonged labor
Rapid labor

point between the time of delivery and up to 12 weeks post-delivery [1]. A common ED presentation of PPH is after a second or third trimester abortion, whether spontaneous or induced. Others may present after the delivery of a viable fetus, either at home or at a stand-alone medical facility.

The most common cause of PPH is uterine atony (70% of cases), followed by trauma (20% of cases) and retained placenta (10% of cases) [10]. Coagulopathies are a rare cause of PPH (1% of cases) [10]. The approach to treatment must be tailored to address the suspected cause.

Though less helpful in the emergency setting, there are risk factors to determine which patients are more likely to experience PPH (Table 13.7).

History and Physical Exam

When evaluating a postpartum patient with bleeding, the priority is to determine stability through a rapid and targeted history and physical. History should be utilized to first evaluate for symptoms of hypovolemia, including lightheadedness, shortness of breath, weakness, syncope, confusion, and blurry vision. Second, the history can help localize the source of bleeding (gynecologic or non-gynecologic). Lastly, history may help identify reversible causes for bleeding such as coagulopathy due to medications or genetic disorder.

The initial focus of the physical exam should be on assessing the airway, breathing, and circulation (ABCs). Particular attention should attempt to identify signs of hemodynamic compromise, hypovolemia, and anemia: pallor, cool or clammy skin, delayed capillary refill, lethargy, confusion, or agitation.

Upon initial evaluation of a patient with PPH, the resuscitation team should obtain a full set of vital signs. Though an essential component of the evaluation, vital signs must be interpreted with a critical eye in pregnant and postpartum women experiencing bleeding. Maternal physiology undergoes significant adaptation during pregnancy, including increased blood volume, increased cardiac output, and decreased systemic vascular resistance, to nurture the growing fetus and to offer protection from the untoward effects of bleeding experienced during delivery. As a result, these patients can compensate for blood loss extensively without demonstrating typical signs of hemorrhagic shock.

Patients who have lost 10–15% of their blood volume (500–1000 mL) may display mild tachycardia and experience lightheadedness and palpitations; however, their blood pressure will remain within normal limits. Patients who have lost 15–25% of their blood volume (1000–1500 mL) will demonstrate an increase in heart rate (110–120 beats/minute) and may experience weakness and sweating and feel unwell. They may also display decreased blood pressure at this point, though their systolic blood pressure will likely remain above 90 mmHg. Patients who have lost 25–35% of their blood volume (1500–2000 mL) may develop more notable tachycardia (120–140 beats/minute) and will finally display significant hypotension (systolic blood pressure less than 90 mmHg). With the significant blood loss, cerebral and peripheral perfusion may be compromised, leading to restlessness, pallor, and/or confusion [3]. Patients with preeclampsia or hypertension will have higher baseline blood pressures during pregnancy. Therefore, the change from baseline blood pressure to blood pressure measured during acute hemorrhage may be a more valuable data point than the measurement during the hemorrhage alone.

After evaluating the patient's airway, respiratory, and circulatory status, a brief assessment should be performed to rule out other non-gynecologic sources of bleeding (e.g., rectal, urinary, or perineal). Once a gynecologic source appears to be most likely, a more detailed history and exam can be performed to localize the source of bleeding (vaginal, cervical, or uterine) and the cause [1].

A sterile vaginal speculum exam should be attempted to evaluate for tears or other injury of the vaginal wall, cervix, and sulcus. Ringed forceps may be useful to aid in the evaluation.

Intervention should not be delayed for a patient with PPH and hemodynamic compromise in an attempt to obtain a full history and physical exam. All history, physical, and interventions should be attempted rapidly and, in many cases, simultaneously to prevent life-threatening sequalae of hemorrhage.

Laboratory Studies

Laboratory studies should not drive the initial resuscitation. If an intervention is required, no laboratory test should preclude the intervention. However, lab studies may help identify additional beneficial interventions and assist in trending a patient's course and progress.

Initial labs to evaluate include the items listed and should be repeated every 30 minutes during resuscitation (excluding the type and screen):

Type and Screen Patients with postpartum hemorrhage are likely to require blood transfusion. If the patient's clinical condition allows the time, type and crossmatched blood should be administered. However, in a hemodynamically unstable bleeding patient, type O negative blood should be given with verbal consent if the patient is lucid.

Complete blood count (CBC) including hemoglobin, hematocrit, and platelet counts. Because blood and plasma levels take time to equilibrate during acute hemorrhage, the initial CBC will often frame a less worrisome picture of the patient's status. However, a reassessment of the CBC will provide a trend in values, which may be more useful than a singular CBC.

Disseminated intravascular coagulation (DIC) profile including prothrombin time (PT), partial thromboplastin time (PTT), International Normalized Ratio (INR), fibrinogen, and D-dimer levels. PPH activates disseminated intravascular coagulopathy, and coagulopathy can also exacerbate PPH. The results of these tests, particularly the fibrinogen, may guide clotting factor replacement therapy.

Blood Gas and Lactic Acid Serum pH, bicarbonate, and lactic acid can all be used to monitor progress of resuscitation in patients in shock and are helpful to trend during resuscitation [4].

Ionized Calcium Patients receiving blood transfusions are at risk of developing hypocalcemia, due to chelation of calcium by the citrate contained in administered blood products.

Imaging Findings

Imaging does not play a role in the acute evaluation or acute management of postpartum hemorrhage.

Management

The critical components in the management of a patient with PPH are to stop ongoing bleeding and to replace lost volume. A stepwise approach to accomplish these goals is recommended (Fig. 13.2).

Intravenous Access Obtain at least two large-bore (16G or larger) points of intravenous (IV) access. Place an intraosseous line in any unstable patients for whom IV access cannot be immediately secured.

Deliver the Placenta **(if placenta has not yet been delivered)** First, apply a surgical clamp to the umbilical cord. Place one hand on the uterine fundus (externally), holding the uterus in a fixed position. Then, apply slow, gentle, consistent traction upon the umbilical cord until the placenta emerges from the vagina [5]. Slowly rotate the placenta in a circle to fully remove membranes and reduce the risk of tearing. Be sure to examine the placenta for missing segments which may suggest retained placenta.

Fig. 13.2 Stepwise approach to management of postpartum hemorrhage

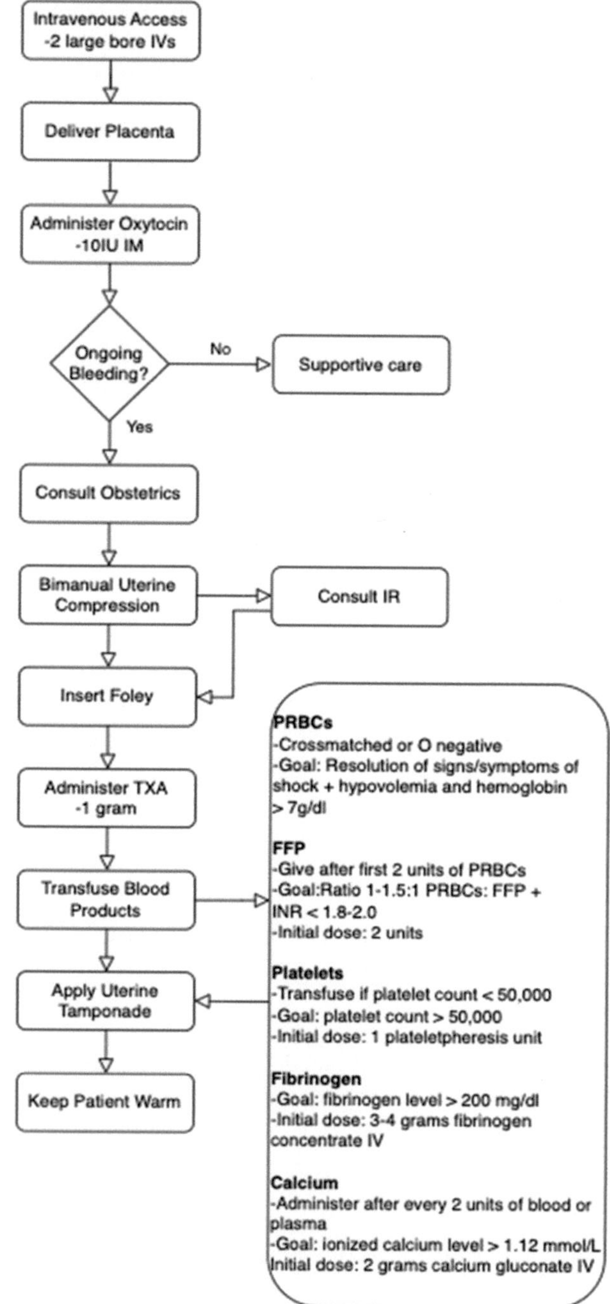

Administer Oxytocin Oxytocin is the most widely used and first choice uterotonic drug (promotes contraction of the uterus). At low doses, oxytocin promotes rhythmic contractions, as in labor, but at higher doses it can cause stronger sustained uterine contractions, which can reduce bleeding from a potentially atonic uterus. Oxytocin should be given either intramuscularly (10 U) [6] or by IV infusion (40 U in one liter of isotonic fluid). 250 mL should infuse over 15 minutes, then the rate of infusion should be titrated based on the rate of ongoing bleeding. If the bleeding remains brisk, the rate should be maintained at 1L/hour, however, if the bleeding slows the rate may be turned down [7]. A large bolus of oxytocin should not be given intravenously due to the risk of hypotension.

If hemorrhage persists despite resuscitation efforts, a second uterotonic agent can be considered (Table 13.8).

External Uterine Massage and Bimanual Uterine Compression The clinician places the non-dominant hand on the patient's abdomen at the fundus and begins a firm massage of the uterus. The dominant hand, wearing a sterile glove, should be inserted into the patient's vagina through the 4Rcervical opening [3]. If any blood clots or retained placenta are palpated, they should be removed from the vagina and/or uterus. Place the dominant hand in the vagina, against the anterior wall of the uterus and make a fist. Pushing against the external hand which has remained on the fundus, compress the uterus between the intra-vaginal hand and the extra-vaginal hand (Fig. 13.3). Maintain this technique of compression while other interventions are being performed until the uterus becomes firm and bleeding has ceased (often at least 8–10 minutes) [11].

Insert a Foley Catheter Bladder decompression improves the uterus's ability to contract [3].

Administer Tranexamic Acid (TXA) TXA reduces bleeding by inhibiting the breakdown of fibrin clots and has been shown to reduce mortality in patients with postpartum hemorrhage [13]. Dosing is 1 g TXA over 10 minutes IV. It is most

Table 13.8 Uterotonic agents for postpartum hemorrhage [6]

Uterotonic agents for postpartum hemorrhage		
Agent	Initial dose	Contraindications
Methylergonovine	0.2 mg intramuscular injection	Hypertension and preeclampsia [3]
Carboprost	0.25 mcg intramuscular injection	Asthma, liver disease, hypertension [3]
Misoprostol	600–1000 mcg by mouth, rectally, or sublingually	Hypersensitivity to misoprostol [3]

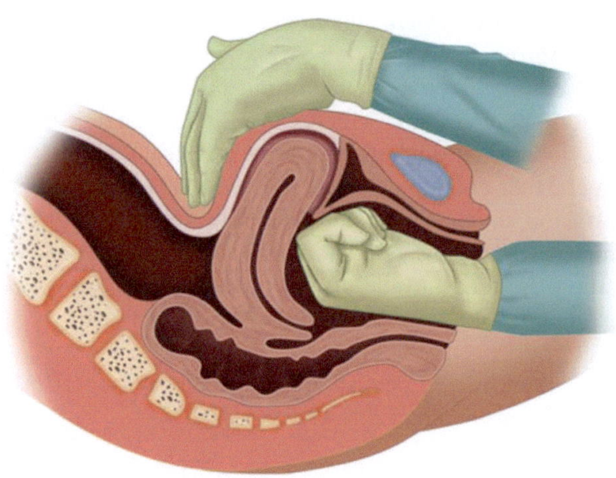

Fig. 13.3 External uterine massage and bimanual uterine compression

effective for patients within 3 hours of delivery [13]. If bleeding persists after 30 minutes, another 1 g dose can be given.

Transfuse Blood Products The decision to transfuse must be based on the clinical assessment of the patient and depends on a number of factors including [14]:

- Presence of clinical features of hypoperfusion.
- The rate of ongoing bleeding.
- Response to medical and surgical interventions enacted.
- The likelihood of continued blood loss.

Blood transfusion strategies in patients with ongoing signs of hypovolemia should aim to attain a ratio between 1 and 1.5:1 of packed red blood cells (PRBCs) to fresh frozen plasma (FFP). Transfusion of platelets is more controversial and can be done empirically as part of a fixed ratio transfusion protocol (e.g., 6 units PRBCs, 4 units FFP, 1 plateletpheresis unit) or in a goal-directed manner if lab data is promptly available [14]. If available, consider utilizing a hospital massive transfusion protocol. Whole blood transfusion strategies are being employed for other hemorrhagic shock states and have shown promising results in the trauma setting [15]. Data on whole blood transfusion in postpartum hemorrhage is limited at this time, and further studies to evaluate efficacy and safety are necessary before this strategy can be recommended [10].

Packed Red Blood Cells help the body maintain intravascular volume and improve oxygen-carrying capacity. Transfusing crossmatched PRBCs is preferred, however O negative blood should be the default blood type used if the urgency for blood administration outpaces the time to properly crossmatch and prepare blood. A patient in shock may require several units of PRBCs. The goal is to attain a hemoglobin greater than 7 g/dL (or hematocrit greater than 0.21%) or resolution of signs/symptoms of shock and hypovolemia [7].

Fresh Frozen Plasma contains the coagulation factors necessary to facilitate the normal clotting cascades. FFP should be given to maintain a 1–1.5:1 ratio of PRBCs to FFP in patients with ongoing signs of shock, hypovolemia, or hemorrhage. Because early administration of FFP has been linked with improved outcomes in hemorrhage, it is recommended to give FFP after the first 2 units of PRBCs have been transfused [16]. The initial dose of FFP is 2–4 units. The goal of FFP administration is an INR less than 1.8–2.0.

Platelets are not described regularly in resuscitation for hemorrhagic shock because data supporting the benefit of empiric platelet transfusion in PPH is not clear. Functioning platelets are necessary for thrombus formation. Indications for platelet transfusion would be to replace poorly functioning platelets (e.g., a patient taking an anti-platelet agent or who has cirrhosis, blood cancer, renal disease, systemic lupus erythematosus, etc.). Currently, experts recommend utilizing lab values (platelet counts <50,000 × 10^9/L) to trigger the transfusion of platelets. The initial dose of platelets is 1 plateletpheresis unit (or 6–8 single donor platelet units, colloquially known as a "six-pack"). The transfusion goal is to attain a platelet count >50,000 × 10^9/L [17].

Fibrinogen is indicated if there is a known fibrinogen deficiency (level < 200 mg/dL) [18] or if a patient is receiving a massive volume transfusion. FFP contains lower concentrations of fibrinogen. Cryoprecipitate has variable concentrations of fibrinogen as well, making dosing difficult. Cryoprecipitate should also be O negative as ABO compatibility is required. Fibrinogen concentrate allows for standardized fibrinogen content and accurate dosing with low infusion volume without concern for ABO compatibility. Initial dosing of fibrinogen concentrate is 3–4 grams IV, which typically increases the fibrinogen level by approximately 100 mg/dL [19]. The goal fibrinogen level is >200 mg/dL [20].

Calcium administration needs to be considered with high volume transfusion resuscitation. PRBCs and FFP contain the anticoagulant citrate which binds calcium and can lead to hypocalcemia in massive transfusion, which in turn can lead to further coagulopathy [21]. In these cases, begin with 2 grams calcium gluconate for every 2 units of blood or plasma administered [22]. The goal marker for calcium resuscitation is an ionized calcium level > 1.12 mmol/L.

Whole blood transfusion is an option for obstetric hemorrhage. The greatest benefit of utilizing whole blood, when available, is a "balanced transfusion" wherein all factors and elements of normal human blood are administered in one transfusion. There is a risk of potential alloimmunization, however, having extracted data from traumatic hemorrhage and limited obstetric hemorrhage publications, and thus its safety in PPH remains unclear [23].

Uterine Tamponade Tamponade is an option to cease PPH particularly when personnel are not available for continuous external uterine massage and bimanual compression. Evidence of efficacy for uterine balloon tamponade is mixed. Patients who continue to bleed despite utilizing other measures should undergo this procedure in

1.	Hold the cervical lip with ringed forceps and apply traction to align the cervical canal and the uterine cavity.
2.	Use forceps to guide the deflated balloon through cervix.
3.	Place the balloon as high in the uterus as possible by applying gentle pressure.
4.	Confirm the position of the balloon with transabdominal ultrasound.
5.	Fill balloon with warm sterile solution until slight resistance to filling is noted and bleeding stops.
6.	Add another 100 mL of sterile solution to keep the balloon in place.
7.	Pack the vagina with moist sterile gauze to prevent retraction of the balloon

Fig. 13.4 Instructions for placing a uterine balloon tamponade Uterine balloon tamponade can be performed with commercial devices or can be modified for limited and low-resource settings [24]

preparation for definitive management (Fig. 13.4) [6]. Balloon tamponade is performed by inserting an inflatable balloon device through the vagina into the uterus then filling it with sterile saline. Commercial devices such as the Bakri [25] and Ebb devices may be available. If not, common hospital supplies may be used to attempt hemostasis (e.g., Foley catheters with 30 cc balloon).

Keep the Patient Warm Patients may experience hypothermia during resuscitation due to administration of room temperature blood products and/or general skin exposure. Hypothermia can negatively affect the coagulation cascade and promote ongoing bleeding [20]. Maintain euthermia by applying passive warming devices and utilizing blood warmers for all transfusions.

Consultation Considerations

Obstetrics should be consulted as soon as postpartum hemorrhage has been identified, to help determine whether surgical intervention is indicated (e.g., arterial ligation, uterine compression sutures, hysterectomy). Obstetricians may also assist with directing or performing interventions for PPH.

Interventional radiology should be consulted for patients who have ongoing hemorrhage after application of bimanual uterine compression and administration of oxytocin to determine if uterine artery embolization may be useful.

Extracorporeal membrane oxygenation (ECMO), a form of life support in which blood is oxygenated outside of the body, augmenting the function of an ailing heart or lungs, has been applied to a small number of PPH patients, with very limited data to support its use [26–28]. However, in patients with shock refractory to the interventions outlined or those who are peri-arrest, a consultation to the ECMO team (if available) should be made to discuss this option.

A patient with PPH will need to be admitted to the hospital to observe for hemodynamic stability. Dependent on the severity of the patient's illness, admission will require monitoring and interventions ranging from simple telemetry to intensive care.

Emergency Department Course and Outcome

The patient received continuous hemodynamic monitoring and was noted to have a heart rate of 125 beats/minute and a blood pressure of 88/64 mmHg. The team obtained two large-bore peripheral IVs and requested a myriad of labs to identify potential reversible causes of hemorrhage. The physician began external uterine massage and proceeded to apply bimanual uterine compression. The bleeding slowed with these interventions. The nurse administered 10 U of intramuscular oxytocin, 1 g of TXA, and placed a foley catheter. The team activated the hospital massive transfusion protocol and called obstetrics for continued management.

Because the patient was in hemorrhagic shock, she received 2 units of uncross-matched type O negative PRBCs followed by 2 units of fresh frozen plasma using a blood warming transfusion device. Despite the transfusion, she remained hypotensive. She was given an additional 2 units of PRBCs as well as 4 grams of calcium gluconate. Lab studies began to return, and her platelet count and fibrinogen levels were adequate, $> 50,000 \times 10^9$/L and > 200 mg/dL, respectively.

On reassessment, the bleeding continued to slow down and a thorough vaginal exam was performed. No signs of trauma were noted to the vagina, cervix, or sulcus, and no intra-vaginal intervention was required. Due to the presence of some ongoing bleeding, she received 0.2 mg of intramuscular methylergonovine. Interventional radiology was consulted for possible uterine artery embolization. By the time the obstetrician reached the bedside, her vital signs had improved; she had a pulse of 110 beats/minute and a blood pressure of 107/82 mmHg, and the bleeding had abated. The patient was admitted to the obstetrics unit with continuous hemodynamic monitoring. Neither interventional radiology nor obstetrics determined that she would require more aggressive intervention now that she had been medically stabilized. She remained in the hospital for several days, during which time she did not experience any further bleeding. She was discharged home in stable condition.

Key Points

- A preferred definition for postpartum hemorrhage in the emergency setting is "Vaginal blood loss after delivery (any route or timing) leading to hemodynamic instability and/or signs and/or symptoms of hypovolemia [8]."
- Significant tachycardia and hypotension present late in the disease process of postpartum hemorrhage due to the normal physiological changes of pregnancy. As such, any concomitant signs/symptoms of hypovolemia or anemia should be taken seriously.

- Apply a stepwise intervention strategy to optimize hemostasis for postpartum hemorrhage.
- Refractory cases of hemorrhage may benefit from surgical intervention by an obstetrician, or uterine artery embolization performed by an interventional radiologist. However, consultations should be made early in the patient's presentation to allow for the greatest number of options for intervention.

References

1. Committee on Practice Bulletins-Obstetrics. Practice Bulletin No. 183: Postpartum Hemorrhage. Obstet Gynecol. 2017;130(4):e168–86. https://doi.org/10.1097/AOG.0000000000002351.
2. Creanga AA, Berg CJ, Syverson C, Seed K, Bruce FC, Callaghan WM. Pregnancy-related mortality in the United States, 2006-2010. Obstet Gynecol. 2015;125(1):5–12. https://doi.org/10.1097/AOG.0000000000000564.
3. Dethier D, Schantz-Dunn. Postpartum Hemorrhage. In: Dobiesz V, Kerrigan K, editors. Manual of obstetric emergencies. 1st ed. Philadelphia: Lippincott Williams & Wilkins (LWW); 2020. p. 371–81.
4. Kogutt BK, Vaught AJ. Postpartum hemorrhage (PPH): blood product management and massive transfusion. Semin Perinatol. 2019;43(1):44–50. https://doi.org/10.1053/j.semperi.2018.11.008.
5. Brandt M. The mechanism and management of the third stage of labor. Am J Obstet Gynecol. 1936;25:662.
6. WHO recommendations for the prevention and treatment of postpartum haemorrhage. Geneva: World Health Organization; 2012.
7. Evensen A, Anderson JM, Fontaine P. Postpartum hemorrhage (PPH): prevention and treatment. Am Fam Physician. 2017;95(7):442–9.
8. Leduc D, Senikas V, Lalonde AB. No. 235-active management of the third stage of labour: prevention and treatment of postpartum hemorrhage. J Obstet Gynaecol Can. 2018;40(12):e841–55. https://doi.org/10.1016/j.jogc.2018.09.024.
9. Patel S, Rodriguez AN, Macias DA, Morgan J, Kraus A, Spong CY. A gap in care? Postpartum women presenting to the emergency room and getting readmitted. Am J Perinatol. 2020;37(14):1385–92. https://doi.org/10.1055/s-0040-1712170.
10. Morris DS, Braverman MA, Corean J, Myers JC, Xenakis E, Ireland K, Greebon L, Ilstrup S, Jenkins DH. Whole blood for postpartum hemorrhage (PPH): early experience at two institutions. Transfusion. 2020;60(Suppl 3):S31–5. https://doi.org/10.1111/trf.15731.
11. Casanova R, Chuang A. Beckmann and Ling's obstetrics and gynecology, 8e. Wolters Kluwer Health, Inc; 2019.
12. Okunlola O, Raza S, Osasan S, Sethia S, Batool T, Bambhroliya Z, et al. Race/ethnicity as a risk factor in the development of postpartum hemorrhage (PPH): a thorough systematic review of disparity in the relationship between pregnancy and the rate of postpartum Hemorrhage. Cureus. 2022;14(6):e26460. https://doi.org/10.7759/cureus.26460.
13. WOMAN Trial Collaborators. Effect of early tranexamic acid administration on mortality, hysterectomy, and other morbidities in women with post-partum haemorrhage (WOMAN): an international, randomised, double-blind, placebo-controlled trial. Lancet. 2017 May 27;389(10084):2105–2116. https://doi.org/10.1016/S0140-6736(17)30638-4. Erratum in: Lancet 2017 May 27;389(10084):2104.
14. Butwick A, Lyell D, Goodnough L. How do I manage severe postpartum hemorrhage? Transfusion. 2020;60(5):897–907. https://doi.org/10.1111/trf.15794.

15. Hanna K, Bible L, Chehab M, Asmar S, Douglas M, Ditillo M, Castanon L, Tang A, Joseph B. Nationwide analysis of whole blood hemostatic resuscitation in civilian trauma. J Trauma Acute Care Surg. 2020;89(2):329–35. https://doi.org/10.1097/TA.0000000000002753.
16. California Maternal Quality Care Collaborative. Obstetric hemorrhage toolkit, Version 3.0. 2022.
17. Jansen AJG, van Rhenen DJ, Steegers EAP, Duvekot JJ. Postpartum Hemorrhage and Transfusion of Blood and Blood Components. Obstet Gynecol Surv. 2005;60:663–71. https://doi.org/10.1097/01.ogx.0000180909.31293.cf.
18. de Lloyd L, Bovington R, Kaye A, Collis RE, Rayment R, Sanders J, Rees A, Collins PW. Standard haemostatic tests following major obstetric haemorrhage. Int J Obstet Anesth. 2011;20(2):135–41. https://doi.org/10.1016/j.ijoa.2010.12.002.
19. Matsunaga S, Takai Y, Nakamura E, Era S, Ono Y, Yamamoto K, Maeda H, Seki H. The clinical efficacy of fibrinogen concentrate in massive obstetric haemorrhage with Hypofibrinogenaemia. Sci Rep. 2017;24(7):46749. https://doi.org/10.1038/srep46749.
20. Jackson DL, DeLoughery TG. Postpartum hemorrhage (PPH): management of massive transfusion. Obstet Gynecol Surv. 2018;73(7):418–22. https://doi.org/10.1097/OGX.0000000000000582.
21. Ditzel RM Jr, Anderson JL, Eisenhart WJ, Rankin CJ, DeFeo DR, Oak S, Siegler J. A review of transfusion- and trauma-induced hypocalcemia: is it time to change the lethal triad to the lethal diamond? J Trauma Acute Care Surg. 2020;88(3):434–9. https://doi.org/10.1097/TA.0000000000002570.
22. Giancarelli A, Birrer KL, Alban RF, Hobbs BP, Liu-DeRyke X. Hypocalcemia in trauma patients receiving massive transfusion. J Surg Res. 2016;202(1):182–7. https://doi.org/10.1016/j.jss.2015.12.036.
23. Polzin A, Smith K, Rumpza T. Whole blood administration for obstetric-related hemorrhage during prehospital transport. Obstet Gynecol. 2023;142(5):1248–51. https://doi.org/10.1097/AOG.0000000000005320.
24. Uterine Balloon Tamponade ENGLISH. Global Health media accessed may 16, 2024. https://www.merckmanuals.com/professional/multimedia/video/uterine-balloon-tamponade
25. Revert M, Cottenet J, Raynal P, Cibot E, Quantin C, Rozenberg P. Intrauterine balloon tamponade for management of severe postpartum haemorrhage in a perinatal network: a prospective cohort study. BJOG. 2017;124(8):1255–62. https://doi.org/10.1111/1471-0528.14382.
26. Huang KY, Li YP, Lin SY, Shih JC, Chen YS, Lee CN. Extracorporeal membrane oxygenation application in post-partum hemorrhage patients: is post-partum hemorrhage contraindicated? J Obstet Gynaecol Res. 2017;43(10):1649–54. https://doi.org/10.1111/jog.13426.
27. Zhang JJY, Ong JA, Syn NL, Lorusso R, Tan CS, MacLaren G, Ramanathan K. Extracorporeal membrane oxygenation in pregnant and postpartum women: a systematic review and meta-regression analysis. J Intensive Care Med. 2021;36(2):220–8. https://doi.org/10.1177/0885066619892826.
28. Ko RE, Chung CR, Yang JH, Jeon K, Suh GY, Oh SY, Choi SJ, Yang JH, Sung K, Cho YH. Use of extracorporeal membrane oxygenation in postpartum patients with refractory shock or respiratory failure. Sci Rep. 2021;11(1):887. https://doi.org/10.1038/s41598-020-80423-w.

Amniotic Fluid Embolism

An Ill-defined Danger

Kiara Rogers

Case

A 38-year-old woman, G4P3, at 39 weeks' gestation arrived at the emergency department (ED) minutes after giving birth. According to emergency medical services (EMS), she was by herself at home when she began having strong contractions approximately one hour before EMS arrived at her home. She hoped she could wait for her husband to return home to accompany her to the hospital, so she waited. Unfortunately, the pain was too intense, so she called for help. By the time EMS arrived, the patient was actively pushing. The patient arrived at the emergency department about 3 minutes after spontaneous vaginal delivery facilitated by emergency medical technicians. The umbilical cord was clamped and cut. Per EMS, the patient had the following vital signs en route:

- Heart rate: 110 beats/minute
- Blood pressure: 119/84 mmHg
- Oxygen saturation: 99% on room air
- Respiratory rate: 14 breaths/minute

On arrival, the obstetrics team was paged and members promptly arrived at the patient's bedside. Because the patient was actively delivering the placenta, the team decided to continue to facilitate delivery in the ED and started oxytocin. While awaiting transport to the labor and delivery unit, the patient suddenly became short of breath, sweaty, and overall ill-appearing, exhibiting marked changes in vital signs and appearing in severe distress.

K. Rogers (✉)
Department of Emergency Medicine, McGovern School of Medicine, University of Texas Health Sciences Center at Houston, Houston, TX, USA

A. A. Kosoko (ed.), *Emergency Medicine Case-Based Guide*,
https://doi.org/10.1007/978-3-031-70118-4_14

"

- Past medical history: Mild persistent asthma
- Past surgical history: Tonsillectomy
- Medications: Albuterol inhaler
- Allergies: Seasonal
- Family history: Mother has hypertension
- Social history: Married. No tobacco or drug use. Social alcohol use prior to pregnancy.

Physical Exam

- Vital signs
  - Heart rate: 153 beats/minute.
  - Blood pressure: 77/43 mmHg
  - Respiratory rate: 38 breaths/minute
  - Temperature: 98.7 °F
  - Oxygen saturation: 84% on room air
- General appearance: Ill appearing, acute distress, diaphoretic
- HEENT
  - Head: Normocephalic, atraumatic
  - Eyes: Normal
  - Ears: Normal
  - Nose: Normal
- Heart: Tachycardia, no murmurs, weak peripheral and central pulses
- Lungs: Tachypnea, retractions, actively attempting to sit forward in bed, diffuse rales on auscultation
- Abdominal/GI: Distended abdomen with palpable boggy uterus.
- Genitourinary: Slow bleeding from vagina
- Extremities: No swelling or deformity
- Neuro: Slightly confused and agitated, moving all extremities
- Skin: No rashes, oozing blood around intravenous line (IV) insertion site

Pertinent Diagnostic Tests (Figs. 14.1 and 14.2, Tables 14.1, 14.2, 14.3, 14.4, 14.5 and 14.6)

Learning Points

Background

Amniotic fluid embolism (AFE) is a rare, but serious, cause of maternal syncope or cardiovascular failure either during labor or shortly after delivery. It is possible during other stages of pregnancy when the amniotic fluid is at risk for entering maternal

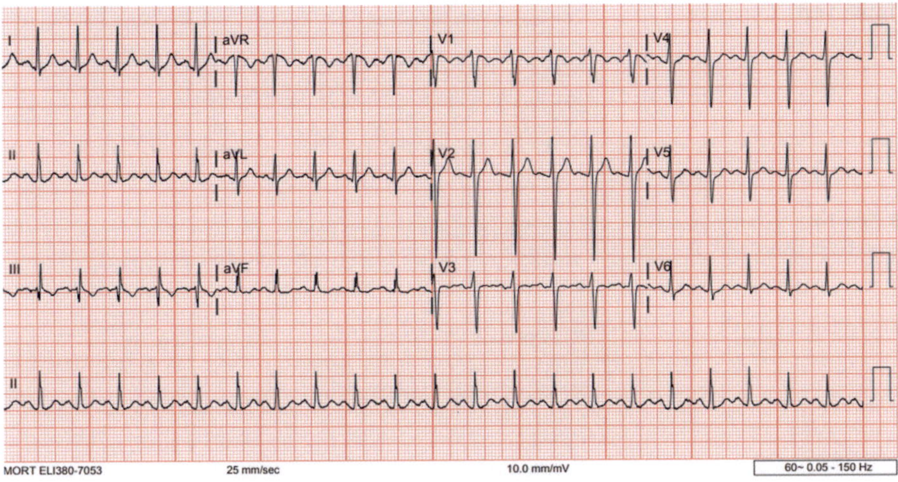

Fig. 14.1 Electrocardiogram (ECG): Sinus tachycardia. Non-specific ST/T-wave abnormality. (Author's own image)

Fig. 14.2 Chest radiograph (CXR): Pulmonary edema with small bilateral pleural effusions. An endotracheal tube is in place with the tip above the carina. (Author's own image)

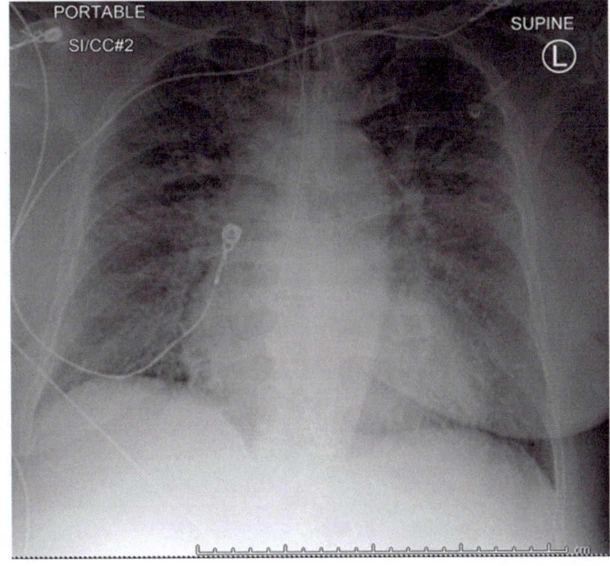

circulation (e.g., induced abortions, surgical trauma, transabdominal amniocentesis) [1]. AFE is usually a diagnosis of exclusion. Unfortunately, it can mimic other serious pathologies. AFE should be suspected when there is evidence of sudden cardiovascular collapse, hypoxia/respiratory failure, seizures, and/or coagulopathy. If not recognized early, AFE can cause catastrophic outcomes for the mother, fetus, or both.

Table 14.1 Complete blood count

Complete blood count	
White blood cells	16.5×10^9/L
Hemoglobin	7.6 g/dL
Hematocrit	22.8%
Platelets	98x $\times 10^9$/L

Table 14.2 Comprehensive metabolic panel

Comprehensive metabolic panel	
Sodium	130 mEq/L
Potassium	4.2 mEq/L
Chloride	110 mEq/L
Bicarbonate	22 mEq/L
Glucose	115 mg/dL
Blood urea nitrogen (BUN)	46 mg/dL
Creatinine	2.6 mg/dL
Calcium	9.6 mg/dL
Total bilirubin	1.2 mg/dL
Alkaline phosphatase	200 units/L
Aspartate aminotransferase (AST)	35 units/L
Alanine aminotransferase (ALT)	25 units/L
Albumin	4.0 g/dL
Total protein	7.1 g/dL

Table 14.3 Venous blood gas and lactic acid

Venous blood gas and lactic acid	
pH	7.23
pCO2	55 mmHg
pO2	25 mmHg
HCO3	23 mEq/L
Lactic acid	5.6 mEq/L

Table 14.4 Coagulopathy panel

Coagulopathy panel	
International normalized ratio (INR)	1.8
Prothrombin time (PT)	31 seconds
Activated partial thromboplastin time (aPTT)	63 seconds

Table 14.5 D-Dimer

D-Dimer	>500 ng/mL

Table 14.6 Fibrinogen

Fibrinogen	95 mg/dL

Though the name "amniotic fluid embolism" induces a mental image of a physical obstruction of maternal circulation due to amniotic fluid particles, this is rarely, if ever, the case. Since amniotic fluid can be dissolved in blood and any other fetal tissue or debris in the amniotic fluid that is introduced into maternal circulation is likely too small to cause significant vascular obstruction alone, newer theories regarding the pathophysiology of AFE have been adopted [2]. More recently, AFE is considered a severe systemic inflammatory process in which the maternal inflammatory system is activated by contents of the amniotic fluid. The details of this inflammatory response are ill-defined. However, a current hypothesis is that some women experience activation of inflammatory mediators which then cause a systemic response akin to a distributive shock comparable to anaphylaxis or sepsis [3, 4]. Nonetheless, researchers agree that for this condition to occur, maternal circulation must receive a significant influx of fetal (amniotic) components *and* a significant immune/anaphylactoid reaction must be mounted against those fetal components [5]. Research has not identified precisely why this reaction occurs in certain women. There are even multiple pathology reports describing fetal cellular debris identified in maternal circulation in cases unrelated to a diagnosis AFE. Interestingly, these findings were identified in patients who lacked clinical features or diagnoses of AFE [3].

The current physiologic theory is that after the release of inflammatory mediators, the initial maternal response is pulmonary vasospasm and vasoconstriction, which then leads to right ventricular failure. This subsequently causes not only respiratory failure, but also eventual left heart failure [6, 7]. Additionally, it is thought that the amniotic fluid itself may cause the activation of the clotting cascade and precipitates a coagulopathy (typically disseminated intravascular coagulopathy, DIC), leading to further hemodynamic instability. This can be immediate or delayed in onset [7].

Differential Diagnosis Pulmonary thromboembolism, air embolism, myocardial infarction, anesthetic complications, anaphylaxis, septic shock, drug-induced allergic reaction, postpartum hemorrhage, uterine rupture, eclampsia, placental abruption, transfusion reaction.

History and Physical Exam

The primary history and exam findings of an amniotic fluid embolism are those that indicate active or impending cardiorespiratory collapse. The classic clinical triad of hypotension, sudden hypoxia, and coagulopathy would highly suggest AFE. However, all three traits are not necessary for diagnosis. Patients may complain of shortness of breath, chest pain, or feelings of anxiety. Physical exam findings can include respiratory distress, tachypnea, tachycardia, agitation, and/or confusion. Signs of coagulopathy, such as excessive or uncontrolled vaginal bleeding, uterine atony, or bleeding from venipuncture sites or cesarean section incisions, may also be prominent features in patients with AFE. If amniotic fluid embolism occurs prior to delivery, there may also be signs of fetal distress captured on continuous fetal monitoring.

Experts have developed criteria for the diagnosis of amniotic fluid embolism [8]. However, it should be noted that these criteria were developed for *research* reporting of AFE and may not correlate completely with clinical practice.

1. Sudden onset of cardiorespiratory arrest. Or, both hypotension (systolic blood pressure < 90 mmHg) and respiratory compromise (dyspnea, cyanosis, or peripheral capillary oxygen saturation < 90%) occurring together.
2. Documentation of apparent DIC following using the scoring system of the Scientific and Standardization Committee on DIC of the International Society on Thrombosis and Hemostasis, modified for pregnancy. Coagulopathy must be detected prior to significant blood loss which itself could account for intravascular dilution or shock-related consumptive coagulopathy.
3. Clinical onset of symptoms during labor or within 30 minutes of delivery of placenta.
4. No fever during labor

Laboratory Studies

There is no specific lab test used to diagnose amniotic fluid embolism. However, there are some critical studies which help guide a physician's management of a patient with AFE. On a complete blood count, there may be an elevated white blood cell count. If DIC is present, then the hemoglobin and hematocrit are expected to be low, secondary to hemorrhage. Furthermore, as expected with DIC, prolonged prothrombin (PT) and partial thromboplastin (PTT) times are expected, in addition to decreased fibrinogen and platelets, and elevated D-dimer. Venous or arterial blood gases may show acidosis (with hypoxemia on an arterial blood gas). There is typically some degree of circulatory shock, and the patient may have elevated lactate. Serum cardiac markers can also increase reflecting cardiac stress or failure [1]..

Imaging Findings

Electrocardiograms may show tachycardia, acute ST and/or T wave changes, or other nonspecific changes in the presence of cardiac strain and/or ischemia. Patients can also develop arrhythmias ranging from subclinical to fatal.

Chest radiograph (CXR) will often demonstrate pulmonary edema or congestion, though CXR might be normal in the early disease stages.

Point-of-care cardiac ultrasound can identify right ventricular or atrial dilation, bowing of the interventricular septum, depressed ejection fraction, or other signs of heart failure. Pulmonary ultrasound may confirm pulmonary edema (interstitial edema) with B-lines.

Management

The mainstay of emergency management of amniotic fluid embolism is supportive. Efforts should focus on resuscitation and stabilization of the patient for whom AFE is suspected prior to handing off care to a differently equipped care environment. The initial goal should be stabilization of any hemodynamic instability. For patients in cardiac arrest, typical measures of immediate cardiopulmonary resuscitation (CPR) and advanced cardiac life support should be attempted. If a cardiac arrest occurs in a gravid patient, rapid delivery (i.e., perimortem cesarian section) should be strongly considered based on gestational age and resources available. Typical post-cardiac arrest care should be initiated early after return of spontaneous circulation.

Both non-invasive and invasive measures should be taken as necessary to provide respiratory support for hypoxia and respiratory distress. Blood pressure and cardiac output support can be enhanced with vasopressors, pulmonary vasodilators, and inotropic medications, keeping in mind that a segment of this population will have right heart dysfunction and excess fluids can be detrimental. Circulatory support cannot be optimized without controlling any significant hemorrhage and correcting coagulopathy. Massive transfusion of blood products may be required. Persistent uterine bleeding because of uterine atony is one source of significant blood loss for any obstetric patient who is actively delivering or who has recently delivered. Oxytocin is typically the first-line medication available and used for uterine hemorrhage.

More advanced treatments that can be considered in refractory cases of AFE will typically need to be performed by a surgeon or interventional radiologist: hysterectomy, uterine artery ablation, intra-aortic balloon counterpulsation (pump). Patients with severe symptoms of AFE may be candidates for emergency extracorporeal membrane oxygenation (ECMO) if experiencing refractory shock. Other invasive efforts could include exchange transfusions or hemodialysis to correct acidosis and potentially to filter the blood of any amniotic fluid and active cytokines [1].

Consultation Considerations

The Society for Maternal Fetal Medicine supports and recommends a multidisciplinary team approach to the care of patients with AFE [7]. This includes early involvement of critical care physicians, maternal fetal medicine services, respiratory therapy, and anesthesiology, if needed.

Obstetrics, particularly those versed in maternal-fetal medicine should be involved early in the patient course, particularly if the patient is actively delivering or the patient is recently postpartum. Specifically, obstetric teams will be able to offer fetal monitoring, but more broadly, they will consider the available and best interventions for positive outcomes for the fetus and the mother. Moreover, a trained obstetrician will be able to intervene with a cesarean section delivery as indicated or even resuscitative hysterectomy in the case of refractory uterine hemorrhage.

Cardiology consultants may assist with the management of cardiogenic shock or decompensated heart failure. They may offer interventions including ECMO or an intra-aortic balloon pump.

At a resource-limited environment, a general surgeon could potentially be another resource for insertion of an intra-aortic balloon pump or other interventions for hemostasis for the hemodynamically unstable patient with suspected AFE. An interventional radiologist may offer other intravascular therapies.

Patients with AFE will often have complicated hospital courses and require the thoughtful care coordination of a critical care specialist.

Emergency Department Course and Outcome

Despite an IV fluid bolus and noninvasive supplemental oxygen, the patient's clinical status remained tenuous. She was becoming increasingly confused. Bedside cardiac and thoracic ultrasound showed B-lines and a dilated right ventricle. She soon did not have identifiable pulses, and she was unable to be aroused. Advanced cardiac life support was initiated, and the patient was intubated. After four rounds of CPR and having received epinephrine, she regained pulses. A norepinephrine drip was initiated. The team placed an arterial catheter and a central venous catheter.

Sometime during her resuscitation, the placenta separated from the uterus. The bleeding had slowed, but there was indeed persistent vaginal bleeding. Her intravascular catheter insertion sites also demonstrated slow oozing of blood. Intravenous oxytocin was infused to aid in hemostasis at the uterus. Her laboratory studies were concerning for advanced coagulopathy and acute anemia, suspected due to blood loss. Emergency-released blood products were transfused, and the local massive transfusion protocol was initiated. She was then admitted to the intensive care unit where she was given multiple blood product transfusions over the course of the next 24 hours. She ultimately required a resuscitative hysterectomy for postpartum hemorrhage. The patient was eventually weaned from the ventilator and had improvement of her coagulopathy. She was extubated and reunited with her newborn child days after giving birth.

Key Points

- The classic triad for AFE is hypotension, sudden hypoxia, and coagulopathy.
- AFE is thought to largely be a severe anaphylactoid reaction to amniotic components in the bloodstream as opposed to an issue of the physical obstruction of vasculature.
- Severe coagulopathy is a common finding in AFE.
- Treatment for AFE is supportive: pursue adequate oxygenation, hemodynamic stability, and correction of coagulopathy.

References

1. Conde-Agudelo A, Romero R. Amniotic fluid embolism (AFE): an evidence-based review. Am J Obstet Gynecol. 2009;201(5):445.e1–13. https://doi.org/10.1016/j.ajog.2009.04.052. Erratum in: Am J Obstet Gynecol 2010 Jan;202(1):92
2. Moldenhauer, JS. Amniotic Fluid Embolism. Merck Manuals Professional Edition. 2021. https://www.merckmanuals.com/professional/gynecology-and-obstetrics/abnormalities-and-complications-of-labor-and-delivery/amniotic-fluid-embolism. Accessed 01 Feb 2023.
3. Clark SL. Amniotic fluid embolism. Obstet Gynecol. 2014;123(2 Pt 1):337–48. https://doi.org/10.1097/AOG.0000000000000107.
4. Tamura N, Farhana M, Oda T, Itoh H, Kanayama N. Amniotic fluid embolism (AFE): pathophysiology from the perspective of pathology. J Obstet Gynaecol Res. 2017;43(4):627–32. https://doi.org/10.1111/jog.13284.
5. Kanayama N, Tamura N. Amniotic fluid embolism (AFE): pathophysiology and new strategies for management. J Obstet Gynaecol Res. 2014;40(6):1507–17. https://doi.org/10.1111/jog.12428.
6. Rudra A, Chatterjee S, Sengupta S, Nandi B, Mitra J. Amniotic fluid embolism. Indian. J Crit Care Med. 2009;13(3):129–35. https://doi.org/10.4103/0972-5229.58537.
7. Pacheco LD, Saade G, Hankins GD, Clark SL. Amniotic fluid embolism (AFE): diagnosis and management. Am J Obstet Gynecol. 2016;215(2):B16–24. https://doi.org/10.1016/j.ajog.2016.03.012.
8. Clark SL, Romero R, Dildy GA, et al. Proposed diagnostic criteria for the case definition of amniotic fluid embolism in research studies. Am J Obstet Gynecol. 2016;215(4):408–12. https://doi.org/10.1016/j.ajog.2016.06.037.

Postpartum Endometritis

A Creeping Suspicion

15

Adedoyin Adesina and Ciaura Brown

Case

A 28-year-old woman, G1P3, presents with 2 days of lower abdominal pain. The pain is sharp and radiates down to her pelvis. She complains of feeling feverish and reports having a brown-tinged vaginal discharge. She was discharged from the hospital 2 days ago after giving birth to a baby girl by cesarean section 5 days prior. Her daughter weighed 8 pounds and 6 ounces and is still in the neonatal intensive care unit due to fever. Prior to the delivery, the patient experienced labor for several days and eventually required emergency cesarean section (C-section) delivery due to failure of progression of labor and a non-reassuring fetal heart tracing. She denies nausea, vomiting, and diarrhea, though she feels constipated. Her last bowel movement was 2 days ago.

- Past medical history: Type 2 diabetes mellitus
- Past surgical history: C-section
- Medications: Metformin, vitamin D, acetaminophen
- Allergies: No known drug allergies
- Family history: Diabetes mellitus in both mother and father
- Social history: Lives with her husband. Works as a store manager. Drinks 1–2 glasses of wine daily but not while pregnant. Denies tobacco use or illicit drug use.

A. Adesina (✉) · C. Brown
Department of Emergency Medicine, Baylor College of Medicine, Houston, TX, USA
e-mail: adedoyia@bcm.edu

© The Author(s), under exclusive license to Springer Nature Switzerland AG 2024
A. A. Kosoko (ed.), *Emergency Medicine Case-Based Guide*,
https://doi.org/10.1007/978-3-031-70118-4_15

Physical Exam

- Vital signs
  - Heart rate: 123 beats/minute
  - Blood pressure: 110/80 mmHg
  - Respiratory rate: 22 breaths/minute
  - Temperature: 101°F
  - Oxygen saturation: 98% on room air
- General appearance: Ill-appearing, appears stated age, pale, diaphoretic
- HEENT
  - Head: Normocephalic, atraumatic
  - Eyes: 4 mm pupils bilaterally, equal, round, and reactive to light; extraocular movement intact, conjunctival pallor
  - Mouth/Throat: Dry mucous membranes, no erythema
  - Neck: Supple, no lymphadenopathy
- Heart: Tachycardia, no murmurs, rubs, or gallops
- Lungs: Clear and equal bilateral breath sounds. No respiratory distress, no use of accessory respiratory muscles
- Abdominal/GI: Lower abdominal horizontal surgical incision. Sutures intact. Suprapubic tenderness. Mild tenderness at surgical wound. No erythema or purulent discharge.
- Genitourinary: Cervical motion tenderness, malodorous lochia, uterine tenderness, no adnexal tenderness.
- Rectal: Deferred
- Extremities: Full range of motion, non-tender, no edema
- Back: No midline tenderness, no costovertebral angle tenderness
- Neuro: Alert and oriented to person, place, and time. Motor and sensation grossly intact.
- Skin: Warm, dry intact. No rash. C-section wound (see abdominal exam).

Pertinent Diagnostic Tests (Tables 15.1, 15.2, 15.3, 15.4 and 15.5)

Table 15.1 Complete blood count

Complete blood count	
White blood cell	18×10^9/L
Hemoglobin	9.0 g/dL
Hematocrit	27%
Platelets	156×10^9/L

Table 15.2 Comprehensive metabolic panel

Comprehensive metabolic panel	
Sodium	137 mEq/L
Potassium	4.2 mEq/L
Chloride	101 mEq/L
Bicarbonate	27 mEq/L
Glucose	97 mg/dL
Blood urea nitrogen (BUN)	9.2 mg/dL
Creatinine	0.7 mg/dL
Calcium	9.4 mg/dL
Total bilirubin	0.3 mg/dL
Alkaline phosphatase	53 units/L
Aspartate aminotransferase (AST)	30 units/L
Alanine aminotransferase (ALT)	23 units/L
Albumin	4.3 g/dL
Total albumin	7.6 g/dL

Table 15.3 Venous blood gas and lactic acid

Venous blood gas and lactic acid	
pH	7.34
pCO2	45 mmHg
pO2	60 mmHg
HCO3	25 mEq/L
Lactic acid	1.8 mg/dL

Table 15.4 Coagulopathy panel

Coagulopathy panel	
International normalized ratio (INR)	1.0
Prothrombin time (PT)	13.8 seconds
Activated partial thromboplastin time (aPTT)	26.2 seconds

Table 15.5 Urinalysis

Urinalysis	
Color	Straw
Appearance	Clear
Specific gravity	≤ 1.005
pH	6.5
Glucose	Negative
Bilirubin	Negative
Ketones	Negative
Protein	Negative
Leukocyte esterase	2+
Nitrites	Negative
White blood cells (WBC)	15
Red blood cells (RBC)	1+
Squamous epithelial cells	Few

Learning Points

Background

Endometritis is an infection of the inner lining of the uterus. It is the most common cause of postpartum infection, with incidence ranging from 1.3 to 1.9% of women with peripartum infections [1, 2]. This uterine infection can be classified as acute or chronic based on the onset, duration, signs, and symptoms, as well as histopathology results [3]. It can be related to or unrelated to pregnancy. Acute endometritis unrelated to pregnancy is typically due to sexually transmitted infections (STIs) and presents categorically as pelvic inflammatory disease. Chronic endometritis usually implies mild signs and symptoms of inflammation which have lasted at least 30 days. Chronic endometritis is usually not associated with pregnancy and usually lacks symptoms or has mild symptoms. It typically requires a histopathologic review for accurate diagnosis. There is up to a 25-fold increased risk of acute endometritis in patients who experienced a C-section delivery compared to vaginal delivery [4]. Although rare, endometritis can occur after spontaneous pregnancy loss or elective pregnancy termination as well, presenting similarly to postpartum endometritis. Postpartum endometritis is the most common postpartum infection and will be the focus of this chapter.

Endometritis occurs typically because of the migration of lower genital flora into the sterile uterine cavity; however, exposures outside of the genital system can also introduce infection to the system. These organisms preferentially colonize devitalized or injured tissue, which can occur after invasive obstetric procedures performed during the peripartum period. The infection can extend beyond the uterine cavity to include the fallopian tubes (salpingitis) and ovaries (oophoritis) and can occur up to 42 days postpartum [5]. The causative organisms are often polymicrobial and can be both aerobic and anaerobic. Some of the most common organisms identified in the endometrial cultures of patients with postpartum endometritis include: *Streptococcus* spp. (specifically Group B *Streptococcus*, GBS), *Staphylococcus* spp., *Enterococcus*, *Gardnerella vaginalis*, *Peptostreptococcus* spp., *Bacteroides* spp., *Escherichia coli*, *Klebsiella pneumoniae*, *Proteus*, and *Ureaplasma urealyticum* [6, 7]. Some patients may develop a systemic illness resulting in sepsis and/or bacteremia.

The greatest risk factor for postpartum endometritis is the mode of childbirth. Higher rates of infections are seen with the C-section procedure, especially when performed after the onset of labor, with prolonged labor, prolonged rupture of membranes, and multi-fetal gestation [4]. Other risk factors associated with endometritis include repeated cervical exams, invasive fetal or uterine monitoring, assisted-vaginal delivery, manual removal of the placenta, and intraamniotic infection. Prophylactic antibiotics have become the standard of care during cesarean section to temper the risk of endometritis. Maternal factors such as demographics, comorbid conditions, and immune status can also contribute to the possibility of developing endometritis, including low socioeconomic status, young maternal age, diabetes mellitus, severe anemia, obesity, human immunodeficiency virus (HIV) infection, or regional colonization with causative bacteria.

Differential Diagnosis surgical wound infection (C-section, perineum), retained foreign body, retained products of conception, chorioamnionitis, intraabdominal infections.

History and Physical Exam

Patients with acute endometritis commonly present with fever and lower abdominal or pelvic pain. Vaginal discharge or lochia is often present and may or may not be malodorous. Symptoms usually occur within 24–72 hours of delivery. Other non-specific systemic symptoms include chills, malaise, lethargy, headache, nausea, and vomiting.

Physical examination findings may include vital signs suggestive of an infection, such as fever, tachycardia, or even hypotension. However, the absence of these vital sign abnormalities should not exclude the diagnosis of acute endometritis. Patient factors such as medications, immunosuppressive state, endocrinopathies, and other comorbid conditions can serve as confounders to a classic presentation. The classic exam finding suggestive of endometritis is uterine tenderness, typically identified on a bimanual exam. The exam may also reveal an enlarged uterus, suprapubic tenderness, and (foul-smelling) vaginal discharge. If septic shock is present, there may be hypotension, altered mental status, and other signs of hypoperfusion. Any accessible surgical sites should be assessed critically for normal healing, including the cutaneous closure and any vaginal tears.

Diagnosis of endometritis is typically made by history and physical exam of the patient with significant risk factors.

Laboratory Studies

Complete blood count (CBC) with differential should be obtained in all patients with suspected endometritis. An elevation in white blood cell count with neutrophil predominance can be seen in the setting of acute infection. However, it is important to note that leukocytosis postpartum is a frequent normal finding, particularly after C-section. Leukocytosis up to nearly $30 \times 10^3/\mu L$ can develop during the labor process and may be present for several days after delivery has occurred [4]. Additionally, patients presenting shortly after delivery are often anemic due to the increase in plasma volume during pregnancy or potential blood loss during delivery.

Additional labs, such as comprehensive metabolic panel (CMP) to assess creatinine and liver enzymes, as well as lactic acid and venous blood gas, should be obtained to help identify any concomitant inadequate end-organ perfusion or identifiers of an acute abdominal illness. Abnormalities in any of these markers would require further investigation and can help guide resuscitation.

Urinalysis should still be obtained as a part of the initial evaluation to assess for a urinary tract infection, which could cause some similar signs and symptoms. In addition, urine culture and urinalysis may reveal the causative agent of endometritis to be urine bacteria or pyuria due to the translocation of bacteria from the urinary tract to the adjacent reproductive organs.

Blood culture is not routinely indicated in uncomplicated endometritis. However, consideration should be given to obtaining blood cultures before starting antibiotics in patients showing signs of systemic infection (e.g., sepsis, altered mental status, hemodynamic instability, end-organ damage). Blood cultures can be helpful in guiding antimicrobial therapy in patients that fail to respond to first-line therapy [8].

Cervical cultures are not routinely recommended as they are prone to growing normal local bacteria rather than isolating pathologic bacteria. However, if an STI is considered as the cause of endometritis, it may be useful to test for *Chlamydia* or *Gonorrhea*, particularly to also encourage treatment of any sexual partners.

Imaging Findings

Imaging is not routinely used to aid in diagnosis of endometritis because the clinical presentation of the patient is most important. However, if a pelvic ultrasound is obtained, it will show a marked heterogeneous and thickened endometrium suggestive of endometritis. Patients who are not showing clinical improvement despite appropriate antibiotic management may benefit from an ultrasound of the pelvis with Doppler flow studies or computed tomography (CT) with intravenous contrast to exclude other plausible diagnoses or complications of endometritis such as pelvic abscess, wound abscess, retained products, thrombophlebitis, or hematoma.

Management

The mainstay treatment for endometritis is broad-spectrum parenteral antibiotics. Intravenous (IV) antibiotics should be initiated promptly in the emergency setting and continued until the patient has been afebrile for 24 hours and with improving pelvic discomfort.

The first-line regimen for endometritis treatment is clindamycin 900 mg IV every 8 hours plus gentamicin 1.5 mg/kg IV every 8 hours (or 5 mg/kg once a day) [9].

If the patient has a history of GBS, there is suspected *Enterococcus* infection, or if there is no improvement after 48 hours of treatment, ampicillin 2 g every 6 hours or ampicillin-sulbactam 3 g every 6 hours can be added.

When IV antibiotics are not available due to limited resources or other barriers to access, an alternative antibiotic regimen should cover the most likely pathogens. As possible alternatives, a systematic review suggests oral and intramuscular antimicrobial options for early postpartum endometritis (Table 15.6) [10].

Table 15.6 Alternative antimicrobial regimens for endometritis in limited-resourced settings

Antibiotic	Dose	Route	Frequency
Clindamycin and gentamicin	600 mg	Oral	Every 6 hours
	4.5 g	Intramuscular	Daily
Amoxicillin-clavulanic acid	875 mg	Oral	Every 12 hours
Meropenem	500 mg	Intramuscular	Every 8 hours
Imipenem-cilastatin	500 mg	Intramuscular	Every 8 hours
Amoxicillin	500 mg	Oral	Every 8 hours

Consultation Considerations

A physician skilled in obstetrics and/or gynecology (Ob/Gyn) should be consulted for evaluation and management recommendations. The consultant will be critical to successful inpatient management of endometritis, any complications, and for follow-up care once the patient is discharged from the hospital. Patients who do not show improvement in fever and abdominal pain within 48 hours of treatment will require further diagnostic workup and consideration for alternate diagnoses [7].

Emergency Department Course and Outcome

The patient remained hemodynamically stable while in the emergency department. She received an IV fluid bolus, acetaminophen for fever, and morphine for pain. The patient was started on IV clindamycin and gentamicin for antimicrobial coverage against endometritis. The patient was admitted to the Ob/Gyn service for further management.

During the hospital stay, the patient continued to receive scheduled IV antibiotics and she was started on a gentle laxative for her constipation. By hospital day three, the patient was afebrile and the pelvic and abdominal pain had improved. The patient was tolerating a normal diet and having normal bowel movements. The patient was discharged home on hospital day 4 with a prescription for amoxicillin-clavulanate for 6 more days and a plan for an outpatient clinic appointment in the Ob/Gyn clinic in 2 weeks.

Key Points

- A cesarean section delivery or other delivery instrumentalization are the greatest risk factors for postpartum endometritis.
- Endometritis should be a clinical diagnosis based on a postpartum patient with fever and pelvic pain, and perhaps vaginal discharge.
- Routine imaging is not necessary, rather imaging is used to evaluate for a failure to respond to an appropriate antibiotic regimen, in order to evaluate for other

causes of pelvic pain and fever, or to examine for complications of endometritis.

- Clindamycin and gentamicin given IV are first-line therapy for endometritis. Treatment should continue until the patient is afebrile for 24 hours with improving abdominal pain.

References

1. Chaim W, Bashiri A, Bar-David J, Shoham-Vardi I, Mazor M. Prevalence and clinical significance of postpartum endometritis and wound infection. Infect Dis Obstet Gynecol. 2000;8(2):77–82. https://doi.org/10.1002/(SICI)1098-0997(2000)8:2<77::AID-IDOG3>3.0.CO;2-6.
2. Woodd SL, Montoya A, Barreix M, Pi L, Calvert C, Rehman AM, Chou D, Campbell OM. Incidence of maternal peripartum infection: a systematic review and meta-analysis. PLoS Med. 2019;16(12):e1002984. https://doi.org/10.1371/journal.pmed.1002984.
3. Kitaya K, Takeuchi T, Mizuta S, Matsubayashi H, Ishikawa T. Endometritis: new time, new concepts. Fertil Steril. 2018;110(3):344–50. https://doi.org/10.1016/j.fertnstert.2018.04.012.
4. Taylor M, Pillarisetty LS. Endometritis. [Updated 2022 May 8]. In: StatPearls [Internet]. Treasure Island (FL): StatPearls Publishing; 2022 Jan. https://www.ncbi.nlm.nih.gov/books/NBK553124/
5. World Health Organization. WHO recommendations for prevention and treatment of maternal peripartum infections. World Health Organization; 2016 Feb 12.
6. Rosene K, Eschenbach DA, Tompkins LS, Kenny GE, Watkins H. Polymicrobial early postpartum endometritis with facultative and anaerobic bacteria, genital mycoplasmas, and Chlamydia trachomatis: treatment with piperacillin or cefoxitin. J Infect Dis. 1986;153(6):1028–37. https://doi.org/10.1093/infdis/153.6.1028.
7. Moldenhauer JS. Postpartum endometritis - gynecology and obstetrics. Merck Manuals Professional Edition. 14 Dec 2022. Available from: https://www.merckmanuals.com/professional/gynecology-and-obstetrics/postpartum-care-and-associated-disorders/postpartum-endometritis. Accessed 30 Dec 2022.
8. Gibbs R, Bauer M, Olvera L, Sakowski C, Cape V, Main E. Improving diagnosis and treatment of maternal sepsis: a quality improvement toolkit.
9. Mackeen AD, Packard RE, Ota E, Speer L, Cochrane Pregnancy and Childbirth Group. Antibiotic regimens for postpartum endometritis. Cochrane Database Systemat Rev. 1996;2015(12). https://doi.org/10.1002/14651858.CD001067.pub3.
10. Meaney-Delman D, Bartlett LA, Gravett MG, Jamieson DJ. Oral and intramuscular treatment options for early postpartum endometritis in low-resource settings: a systematic review. Obstet Gynecol. 2015;125(4):789–800. https://doi.org/10.1097/aog.0000000000000732.

Mastitis

Is This Heat Curdling My Milk?

Monalisa Muchatuta, Omoefe Ebhohimen,
and Pierre-Carole Tchouapi

Case

A 26-year-old woman, G1P1, presents to the emergency department (ED) complaining of right breast pain, redness, and swelling for 4 days. She delivered her first child 8 days ago after an uneventful pregnancy. She reports breastfeeding the infant exclusively and that it had been going well until this new development with her breast. She reports that her right breast has progressively become more tender and swollen and is now painful to touch, including when she breastfeeds her infant. She has been taking acetaminophen and using a warm compress as suggested by her mother for pain, but the swelling and redness have not resolved. She reports subjective fever and chills at home. She denies trauma to the breast, nausea, vomiting, abdominal pain, recent illness, or unintentional recent weight loss.

- Past medical history: Generalized anxiety disorder
- Past surgical history: None
- Medications: Prenatal vitamins
- Allergies: No known drug allergies
- Family history: Father with hypertension
- Social history: Non-smoker, no illicit drug use, no alcohol

M. Muchatuta (✉) · O. Ebhohimen · P.-C. Tchouapi
Department of Emergency Medicine, State University of New York Downstate Health
Sciences University, Brooklyn, NY, USA
e-mail: monalisa.muchatuta@downstate.edu

© The Author(s), under exclusive license to Springer Nature Switzerland AG 2024
A. A. Kosoko (ed.), *Emergency Medicine Case-Based Guide*,
https://doi.org/10.1007/978-3-031-70118-4_16

Physical Exam

- Vital signs
  - Heart rate: 101 beats/minute
  - Blood pressure: 129/80 mmHg
  - Respiratory pate: 12 breaths/minute
  - Temperature: 101 °F
  - Oxygen saturation: 99% on room air
- General appearance: Well-appearing, no acute distress, appears stated age
- Heart: S1, S2 regular rate and rhythm; no murmurs, rubs, or gallops
- Lungs: Clear lung sounds bilaterally
- Chest: Left breast normal appearing. Right breast engorged, warm and tender to touch, diffuse erythema of areola and approximately 2 cm of surrounding skin tissue, no obvious fluctuance, no expressible purulence
- Abdominal/GI: Soft, nontender, bowel sounds present
- Genitourinary: Normal external exam
- Extremities: Moves all extremities spontaneously
- Neuro: Alert, oriented, motor and sensation intact grossly
- Skin: Normal
- Lymph: Normal
- Psych: Normal

Pertinent Diagnostic Tests (Tables 16.1, 16.2 and 16.3)

Table 16.1 Complete blood count with differential

Complete blood count	
White blood cells	12×10^9/L
Red Blood Cells	4.8×10^{12}/L
Neutrophil	58.0%
Lymphocytes	28.9%
Monocytes	10.7%
Eosinophils	1.5%
Basophils	0.7%
Immature granulocytes	0.2%
Nucleated red blood cells	0%
Hemoglobin	14.7 g/dL
Hematocrit	46.7%
Platelets	205×10^9/L

Table 16.2 Comprehensive metabolic panel

Comprehensive metabolic panel	
Sodium	139 mmol/L
Potassium	4.8 mmol/L
Chloride	102 mmol/L
Bicarbonate	23 mmol/L
Glucose	99 mg/dL
Blood urea nitrogen (BUN)	14 mg/dL
Creatinine	1.0 mg/dL
Calcium	9.2 mg/dL
Total bilirubin	0.5 mg/dL
Alkaline phosphatase	56 units/L
Aspartate aminotransferase (AST)	29 units/L
Alanine aminotransferase (ALT)	24 units/L
Albumin	3.9 g/dL
Total protein	7.3 g/dL

Table 16.3 Venous blood gas and lactic acid

Venous blood gas and lactic acid	
pH	7.42
pCO2	41.8 mmHg
pO2	40.4 mmHg
HCO3	26.9 mEq/L
Lactic acid	1.4 mEq/L

Learning Points

Background

Mastitis is the inflammation or infection (usually bacterial) of the mammary glands in the breasts [1]. Classification of mastitis varies by patient population and can be grouped into two large categories: lactational (puerperal) and non-lactational (non-puerperal) mastitis. Puerperal mastitis is the most common form and typically has infectious etiology in pregnant or lactating women. Non-puerperal mastitis may have infectious, noninfectious, or granulomatous etiology in non-pregnant or lactating people [1, 2].

Mastitis occurs most commonly within the first three weeks (early) postpartum [2]. Breastfeeding or lactating women between the ages of 21 and 35 years [3] are the largest affected demographic, with incidence as high as 33% of early postpartum women [2]. Puerperal mastitis occurs due to stagnant milk in the lactiferous ducts and subsequent bacterial contamination. Stagnant milk in the lactiferous ducts may be due to infrequent feedings, excessive milk supply, a clogged duct, or poor and/or uncoordinated suckling of the child [1]. Bacteria from the feeding baby's mouth or mother's skin are generally introduced to ducts through breaks in the skin at the nipple and areola. Bacteria, particularly *Staphylococcus aureus*, can rapidly replicate in the nutrient rich environment of lactational milk, leading to mastitis [1, 2, 4].

Though typically a benign condition, delayed diagnosis can progress to more severe infections, such as abscesses or sepsis which would require hospitalization and possibly surgical intervention. As such, early diagnosis and treatment are necessary for best outcomes [5].

Differential Diagnosis breast abscess, cellulitis, engorged mammary gland, fibrocystic breast tissue, benign breast cyst, breast cancer.

History and Physical Exam

Mastitis is a clinical diagnosis. History should elicit if a woman is breastfeeding and whether the child is latching to the nipple or whether she is expressing milk for the child to then consume from a bottle. Any lactation difficulty should be noted. Engorgement or report of a clogged duct will often precede the classic localized breast features of fever, erythema, swelling, warmth, and/or tenderness [6–8]. Presentation usually occurs in the first few weeks of breastfeeding postpartum but potentially could occur any time in a breastfeeding woman. Other symptoms may include breast firmness, palpable fluctuance, or chaffed/sore nipples [2, 3, 5]. Mastitis can be a source for sepsis or systemic disease, with patients presenting with myalgias, chills, malaise, or other toxic traits.

Laboratory Studies

No single laboratory test is diagnostic for mastitis. A complete blood cell count (CBC) may show an elevated white cell count or a reactive thrombocytosis but these are nonspecific findings.

It is not common practice to culture breast milk in an ambulatory patient. However, in a septic patient or a patient with refractory symptoms despite antibiotics, cultures may be useful for appropriate antibiotic selection. Nonetheless, skin flora and oral flora are by far the most common culprits for mastitis. Routine evaluation of breast milk cultures may ultimately yield normal flora.

Imaging Findings

Imaging is not routinely indicated when evaluating for mastitis. If there is concern for a breast abscess, an ultrasound is the image of choice. A worsening or non-responsive course despite appropriate antibiotics may suggest formation of an abscess. Less than 10% of mastitis cases develop into an abscess. On ultrasound, an abscess may demonstrate a purulent fluid collection (demarcated hypoechoic area), whereas mastitis may simply have edema of the fatty tissue of the breast [9–12].

Magnetic resonance imaging (MRI) is another option for refractory cases. MRI is not routinely indicated for mastitis but is the most specific of modalities to delineate fluid collection and edema related to breast abscesses versus other diagnoses [9, 10]; MRI is more utilized as a diagnostic modality when evaluating for non-puerperal mastitis than puerperal mastitis [8].

If there is any concern for malignancy, mammography should be obtained as well.

Management

While treatment for non-puerperal mastitis targets the underlying cause [1, 2, 5], supportive measures are the mainstay of therapy for uncomplicated, puerperal mastitis.

Treatment for puerperal mastitis can be divided into two categories: complicated vs. uncomplicated. Most patients with uncomplicated puerperal mastitis will be hemodynamically stable, and generally, treatment will be supportive. However, as should be expected for all patients presenting to the ED, management should initially focus on resuscitation of any hemodynamically unstable septic patient: intravenous fluids, parenteral antibiotics, and antipyretics. Pain is an important presenting complaint for mastitis, which can and should be addressed with analgesics. A provider should be able to coach the patient in addressing the clogged milk ducts which facilitated the subsequent inflammatory processes in the first place. Using warm compresses, simple localized massage, and encouraging expectoration of milk from the nipple should help with forward flow and decrease stasis [13, 14]. Therefore, breastfeeding is generally encouraged despite the infection and inflammation of mastitis [7]. This is helpful to the mother and not harmful to the baby.

Intravenous (IV) or oral (PO) antibiotics are reserved for more serious mastitis infections of the breast [14]. The choice between IV or oral antibiotics depends on whether or not the patient requires admission due to sepsis or hemodynamic instability (Table. 16.4). Antibiotic selection should be sure to target *S. aureus*, *Streptococcus*, and *E. coli*. Most routine cases can be treated with 10–14 days of antibiotics with oral penicillinase-resistant penicillin, cephalosporins, or macrolides (Table 16.5).

For more complex cases requiring inpatient IV administration, preferred antibiotic regimens are 10–14 days, but dependent on suspicion, may also include coverage for methicillin-resistant *S. aureus* (Table 16.5):

If mastitis is clinically diagnosed and a fluid collection is identified by imaging, an abscess is likely. If there is proximity of the abscess to the epidermis (<1 cm depth), the emergency physician can consider performing an incision and drainage

Table 16.4 Oral antibiotic regimens for treating uncomplicated mastitis

Antibiotic	Dose	Frequency
Dicloxacillin [14, 15]	500 mg	Four times daily
Amoxicillin-clavulanate [14]	875–125 mg	Twice daily
Flucloxacillin [2, 13]	500 mg	Four times daily
Cephalexin [14]	500 mg	Four times daily
Clarithromycin [15]	500 mg	Twice daily

Table 16.5 Intravenous antibiotic regimens for treating complicated mastitis

Antibiotic	Dose	Frequency
Nafcillin [15]	2 g	Every 4 hours
Oxacillin [5, 15]	2 g	Every 4 hours
Clindamycin [14, 15]	600 mg	Every 8 hours
Vancomycin [2, 5, 15]	15 mg/kg	Twice daily

(I&D) at bedside based on personal comfort with the procedure (by needle or scalpel). Otherwise, if the fluid collection is deeper (>1 cm depth) from the epidermis, a surgical consult may be necessary to avoid complications of I&D, including cosmetic complications or development of a milk duct fistula. Surgical intervention has become less favorable due to prolonged healing time, interrupted breast feeding, potential poor cosmetic results, and heavy resource requirement [16–18]. It is, however, important to note that abscesses may require multiple needle aspirations for complete eradication of pus [16, 18]. As such, patients will benefit from education and strict return precautions for wound care, with close follow-up to monitor for signs of complications [16–19].

Consultation Considerations

Obstetrician/gynecologist (Ob/Gyn) or primary care outpatient clinic follow-up is most often indicated for patient reassessment. Rarely, is a consultation from the emergency setting necessary [18]. Severe mastitis may take several weeks to fully resolve, but rare cases may progress to a breast abscess. In cases of a breast abscess, a more urgent general surgeon, breast surgeon, or Ob/Gyn consultation should be made.

Several recent studies now recommend the use of ultrasound-guided needle aspiration performed by an interventional radiologist or surgeon adept with using an ultrasound when there is a pathologic significant fluid collection in the breast. This preferred alternative to scalpel or operative drainage cites minimal invasion, reduction in scarring, uninterrupted breastfeeding, and cost effectiveness [16–18].

Emergency Department Course and Outcome

After a thorough history and physical exam, the patient was diagnosed with uncomplicated puerperal mastitis. Her lab studies were reviewed and were not concerning for a more complicated condition. She received 975 mg of oral acetaminophen for pain and fever, and dicloxacillin 500 mg orally. She was discharged with a prescription for a 14-day course of dicloxacillin. She also was coached on supportive care measures to alleviate the mastitis, including use of warm compresses on her breast several times daily and breast massage. She was encouraged to continue breastfeeding her infant or to utilize a breast pump if it would be more comfortable for her.

Three days later, she had a clinic appointment with her primary care provider, where her right breast was noted to be vastly less swollen and less tender. She subsequently completed her antibiotic course prior to a previously scheduled follow-up visit with her Ob/Gyn two weeks later and was found to have complete resolution of her mastitis.

Key Points

- Mastitis can be diagnosed clinically in a breastfeeding person by breast pain associated with swelling, redness, and warmth.
- There is no single clinical lab study which is diagnostic of mastitis, and imaging is rarely indicated.
- A patient with puerperal mastitis should be encouraged to continue breastfeeding or pumping her breast milk as able.
- Oral antibiotics targeting *S. aureus*, *Staphylococcus*, and *E. coli* will often suffice to manage uncomplicated puerperal mastitis along with supportive measures.

References

1. Azer CHS. Puerperal mastitis. In: Elkady A, Sinha P, Hassan SAZ, editors. Infections in pregnancy: an evidence-based approach. Cambridge: Cambridge University Press; 2019. p. 183–5.
2. Boakes E, Woods A, Johnson N, Kadoglou N. Breast infection: a review of diagnosis and management practices. Eur J Breast Health. 2018;14(3):136–43. https://doi.org/10.5152/ejbh.2018.3871.
3. Liu L, Zhou F, Wang P, Yu L, Ma Z, Li Y, et al. Periductal mastitis: an inflammatory disease related to bacterial infection and consequent immune responses? Mediat Inflamm. 2017;2017:5309081. https://doi.org/10.1155/2017/5309081.
4. Zhang Y, Zhou Y, Mao F, Guan J, Sun Q. Clinical characteristics, classification and surgical treatment of periductal mastitis. J Thorac Dis. 2018;10(4):2420–7. https://doi.org/10.21037/jtd.2018.04.22.
5. World Health Organization. Mastitis: causes and management. In: Development DoCaAHa. Geneva: World Health Organization; 2000.
6. Woodard GA, Bhatt AA, Knavel EM, Hunt KN. Mastitis and more: a pictorial review of the red, swollen, and painful breast. J Breast Imaging. 2021;3(1):113–23. Published 9 Dec 2020. https://doi.org/10.1093/jbi/wbaa098.
7. Kent JC, Ashton E, Hardwick CM, Rowan MK, Chia ES, Fairclough KA, et al. Nipple pain in breastfeeding mothers: incidence, causes and treatments. Int J Environ Res Public Health. 2015;12(10):12247–63. https://doi.org/10.3390/ijerph121012247.
8. An JK, Woo JJ, Lee SA. Non-puerperal mastitis masking pre-existing breast malignancy: importance of follow-up imaging. Ultrasonography. 2016;35(2):159–63. https://doi.org/10.14366/usg.15024.
9. Tan H, Li R, Peng W, Liu H, Gu Y, Shen X. Radiological and clinical features of adult non-puerperal mastitis. Br J Radiol. 2013;86(1024):20120657. https://doi.org/10.1259/bjr.20120657.
10. Jari I, Naum AG, Ursaru M, Manafu EG, Gheorghe L, Negru D. Breast infections: diagnosis with ultrasound and mammography. Rev Med Chir Soc Med Nat Iasi. 2015;119(2):419–24.

11. Cheng L, Reddy V, Solmos G, Watkins L, Cimbaluk D, Bitterman P, et al. Mastitis, a radiographic, clinical, and histopathologic review. Breast J. 2015;21(4):403–9. https://doi.org/10.1111/tbj.12430.

12. Yildiz S, Aralasmak A, Kadioglu H, Toprak H, Yetis H, Gucin Z, et al. Radiologic findings of idiopathic granulomatous mastitis. Med Ultrason. 2015;17(1):39–44. https://doi.org/10.11152/mu.2013.2066.171.rfm.

13. Pustotina O. Management of mastitis and breast engorgement in breastfeeding women. J Matern Fetal Neonatal Med. 2016;29(19):3121–5. https://doi.org/10.3109/14767058.2015.1114092.

14. Spencer JP. Management of mastitis in breastfeeding women. Am Fam Physician. 2008;78(6):727–31. Available from: https://www.aafp.org/pubs/afp/issues/2008/0915/p727.html

15. Stevens DL, Bisno AL, Chambers HF, Dellinger EP, Goldstein EJ, Gorbach SL, et al. Practice guidelines for the diagnosis and management of skin and soft tissue infections: 2014 update by the Infectious Diseases Society of America. Clin Infect Dis. 2014;59(2):147–59. https://doi.org/10.1093/cid/ciu444.

16. Egbe TO, Njamen TN, Essome H, Tendongfor N. The estimated incidence of lactational breast abscess and description of its management by percutaneous aspiration at the Douala general hospital, Cameroon. Int Breastfeed J. 2020;15(1):26. https://doi.org/10.1186/s13006-020-00271-2.

17. Kataria K, Srivastava A, Dhar A. Management of lactational mastitis and breast abscesses: review of current knowledge and practice. Indian J Surg. 2013;75(6):430–5. https://doi.org/10.1007/s12262-012-0776-1.

18. Iosifescu S. Mastitis and breast abscesses. EmDOCsnet—Emergency Medicine Education [Internet] 2020. Available from: http://www.emdocs.net/mastitis-and-breast-abscesses/

19. Dixon JM, Khan LR. Treatment of breast infection. BMJ. 2011;342:d396. https://doi.org/10.1136/bmj.d396.

20. Amir LH, AoBMP C. ABM clinical protocol #4: mastitis, revised march 2014. Breastfeed Med. 2014;9(5):239–43. https://doi.org/10.1089/bfm.2014.9984.

Peripartum Cardiomyopathy

It's Getting Harder and Harder to Breathe

Adeola A. Kosoko

Case

A 36-year-old woman, G1P0 at 34 weeks' gestation, is brought in by emergency medical services (EMS) after a syncopal episode while at home. She has had 3 weeks of shortness of breath that acutely worsened today. She has also had lower extremity edema bilaterally. This is the patient's third emergency department visit in this pregnancy. The last visit was 2 weeks ago. These other visits were for feelings of fatigue and shortness of breath. She was reassured by providers each time, having been told that she has been having "expected pregnancy changes." Today, the patient had a syncopal episode upon standing at home. It was witnessed by her mother, who called EMS for help. The episode lasted a few seconds, and the patient is now feeling back to her pregnancy baseline.

- Past medical history: First pregnancy (G1P0) with regular prenatal care, normal prenatal course to date
- Past surgical history: None
- Medications: Prenatal vitamins
- Allergies: No known drug allergies
- Family history: Mother has diabetes
- Social history: Non-smoker, no alcohol, no illicit drug use

Supplementary Information The online version contains supplementary material available at https://doi.org/10.1007/978-3-031-70118-4_17.

A. A. Kosoko (✉)
Department of Emergency Medicine, McGovern School of Medicine, University of Texas Health Sciences Center at Houston, Houston, TX, USA
e-mail: Adeola.A.Kosoko@uth.tmc.edu

Physical Exam

- Vital signs
  - Heart rate: 130 beats/minute
  - Blood pressure: 89/60 mmHg
  - Respiratory rate: 26 breaths/minute
  - Temperature: 99 °F
  - Oxygen saturation: 93% on room air
- General appearance: Appears stated age, sitting up in the bed, in moderate-severe respiratory distress
- HEENT.
  - Head: Atraumatic, normocephalic
  - Eyes: Pupils equal, round, and reactive to light (4–2 mm); external ocular movements are normal; normal conjunctiva; no papilledema
  - Ears: Normal tympanic membranes
  - Nose: Normal
  - Throat: No erythema or edema of the oropharynx
  - Neck: Trachea midline, no stridor, jugular venous distention present
- Heart: Tachycardia, regular rhythm, equal pulses
- Lungs: Moderate respiratory distress, tachypneic, speaks 4- to 5-word sentences, bibasilar rales on auscultation
- Abdominal: Soft, nontender, bowel sounds present, gravid with fundus above the umbilicus
- Genitourinary: Normal external, no vaginal bleeding, internal exam deferred
- Rectal: Normal
- Extremities: 2+ pitting edema in bilateral lower extremities extending to knees, no tenderness, no deformity, tolerates full range of motion, negative Homans' sign bilaterally
- Back: Normal
- Neuro: Alert, oriented, normal reflexes, no clonus
- Skin: Normal
- Lymph: Normal
- Psych: Normal

Pertinent Diagnostic Tests (Figs. 17.1, 17.2, 17.3, 17.4 and 17.5 and Tables 17.1, 17.2, 17.3, 17.4, 17.5, 17.6 and 17.7)

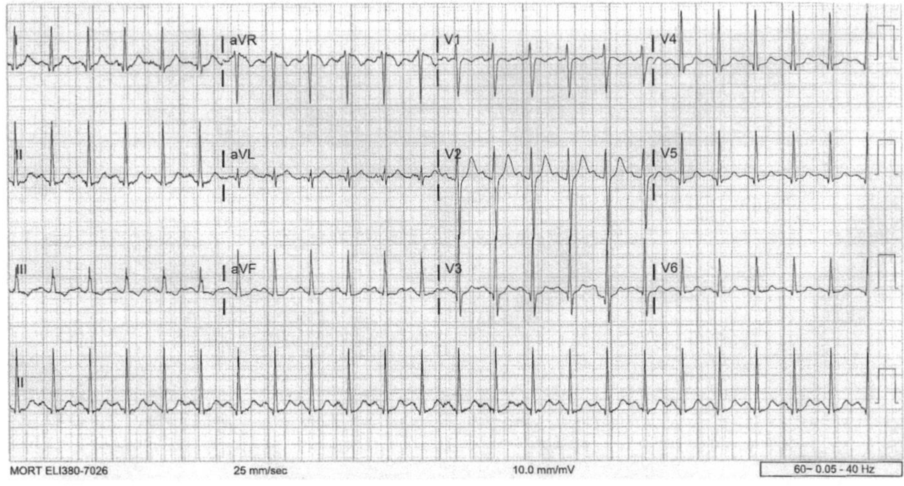

Fig. 17.1 Electrocardiogram (ECG): Sinus tachycardia. Nonspecific T-wave abnormalities. (Author's own image)

Fig. 17.2 Chest radiograph (CXR): Enlarged cardiac silhouette. Pulmonary venous congestion. Cephalization of pulmonary veins. Pulmonary interstitial edema. (Author's own image)

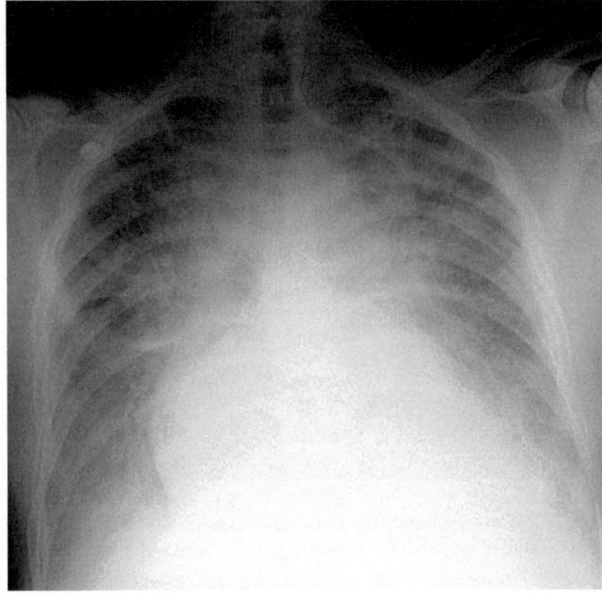

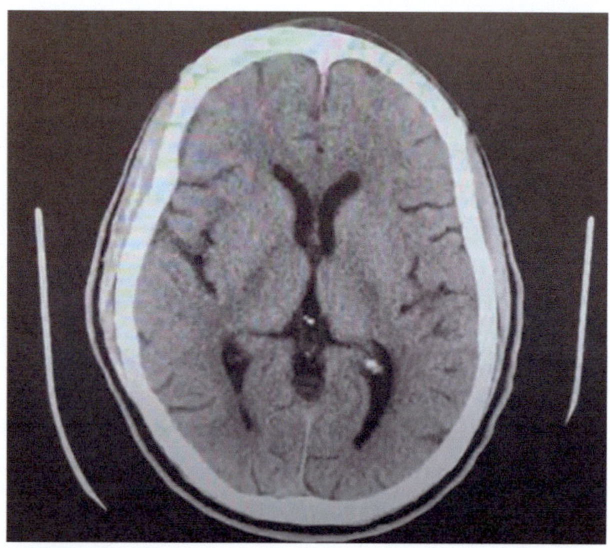

Fig. 17.3 Computer tomography head without contrast (CT head WO): Normal study. (Author's own image)

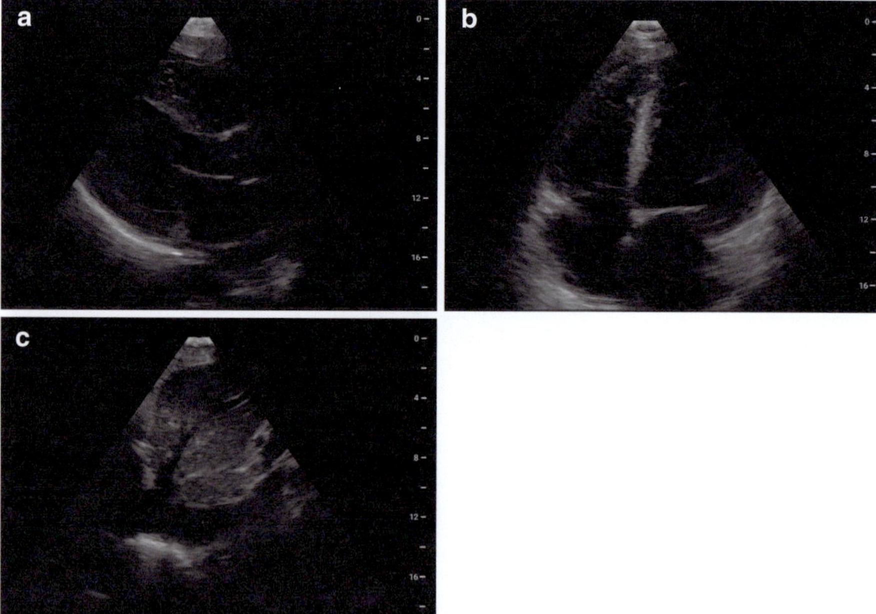

Fig. 17.4 Point-of-care cardiac ultrasound (echocardiogram) (**a**) Parasternal long axis (**b**) apical four-chamber view (**c**) inferior vena cava view: reduced ejection fraction

Echocardiogram exam demonstrating peripartum cardiomyopathy. On the parasternal long axis, there is left ventricular chamber dilation and globally reduced ejection fraction, qualitatively evidenced by poor inward contraction of the endocardial borders of the left ventricle (less than 50% change in chamber size during systole) and minimal movement of the anterior leaflet of the mitral valve toward to interventricular septum. Similarly, the apical four-chamber view demonstrates a globally reduced ejection fraction. The inferior vena cava is dilated with minimal respirophasic variation, indicating high central venous pressure and volume overload with poor forward flow.

Longitudinal images of the bilateral anterior chest wall. Diffuse B-lines Peripartum cardiomyopathy (PPCM) pertinent diagnostic tests diffuse B-lines, defined as hyperechoic, vertical artifacts originating at the pleural lining and extending deep into the lung parenchyma without attenuation, can be seen while scanning the anterior chest in patients with interstitial edema. Three or more B-lines per intercostal space are considered pathologic. In these images, the pulmonary edema is so severe that it appears as almost complete "white-out" of the intercostal space, as the innumerable B-lines coalesce.

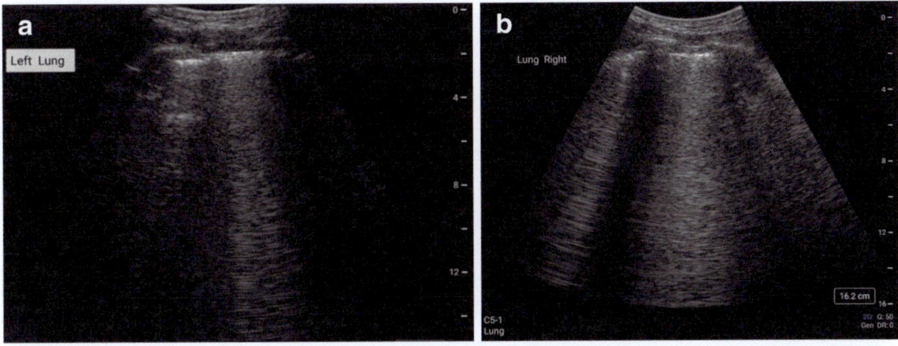

Fig. 17.5 Point-of-care thoracic ultrasound of (**a**) left lung and (**b**) right lung: diffuse B-lines

Table 17.1 Complete blood count

Complete blood count	
White blood cells	15×10^9/L
Hemoglobin	12 g/dL
Hematocrit	36%
Platelets	270×10^9/L

Table 17.2 Comprehensive metabolic panel

Comprehensive metabolic panel	
Sodium	139 mEq/L
Potassium	3.9 mEq/L
Chloride	110 mEq/L
Bicarbonate	26 mEq/L
Glucose	93 mg/dL
Blood urea nitrogen (BUN)	44 mg/dL
Creatinine	1.8 mg/dL
Calcium	9.0 mg/dL
Total bilirubin	0.6 mg/dL
Alkaline phosphatase	60 units/L
Aspartate aminotransferase (AST)	105 units/L
Alanine aminotransferase (ALT)	95 units/L
Albumin	3.6 g/dL
Total protein	6.9 g/dL

Table 17.3 Venous blood gas and lactic acid

Venous blood gas and lactic acid	
pH	7.33
pCO2	25 mmHg
pO2	50 mmHg
HCO3	15 mEq/L
Lactic acid	2.4 mEq/L

Table 17.4 Coagulopathy panel

Coagulopathy panel	
International normalized ratio (INR)	1.13
Prothrombin time (PT)	12.2 seconds
Activated partial thromboplastin time (aPTT)	23.4 seconds

Table 17.5 Troponin I

Troponin I	0.52 ng/mL

Table 17.6 B-Type natriuretic peptide (BNP)

B-type natriuretic peptide (BNP)	829 pg/mL

Table 17.7 Urinalysis

Urinalysis	
Color	Yellow
Appearance	Clear
Specific gravity	1.010
pH	7.0
Glucose	Negative
Bilirubin	Negative
Ketones	0
Protein	1+
Leukocyte esterase	1+
Nitrites	Negative
White blood cells (WBC)	1 WBC/High-Power Field (HPF)
Red blood cells (RBC)	0 RBCs/HPF
Squamous epithelial cells	0–5 cells/HPF

Learning Points

Background

Peripartum cardiomyopathy (PPCM) is an idiopathic cardiomyopathy due to left ventricular (LV) dysfunction during the last month of pregnancy or up to 5 months postpartum. Though LV dilation may not be present, the ejection fraction (EF) is almost always reduced (< 45%). It is a diagnosis that excludes other causes of cardiomyopathy [1, 2].

The definitive pathophysiology of the condition is uncertain. There is a genetic predisposition, which occurs more commonly in certain ethnic groups. A commonly accepted theory suggests that unique time of the peripartum period optimizes hormonal changes (prolactin, tyrosine kinase) that allow for cardiac remodeling [3]. Another theory suggests that vascular insults occur at the peripartum period causing cardiomyopathy [4].

Those at greatest risk for PPCM are described as older than 30 years of age, of African ancestry, or have a history of hypertension, multiparity, malnourishment, and/or smoking [5].

It is important for emergency physicians to be aware of this rare diagnosis because although 50–80% of women with PPCM may eventually recover normal left ventricle systolic function [5], positive outcomes depend on recognition of PPCM as a disease and appropriate management of heart failure.

Differential Diagnosis pulmonary embolism, amniotic fluid embolism, myocarditis, spontaneous coronary artery dissection, acute coronary syndrome, Takotsubo cardiomyopathy, preeclampsia, thyroid disease, normal pregnancy.

History and Physical Exam

Patients usually present with typical heart failure symptoms: dyspnea, peripheral edema, orthopnea, fatigue, palpitations, etc. The patient must be in the peripartum stage to qualify for the diagnosis.

Specifically evaluate for jugular venous distention, peripheral edema, arrhythmia, hypotension to suggest the diagnosis. Advanced disease may present with syncope or cardiogenic shock.

Clinically, a strict diagnosis of PPCM can be made by fulfilling the following criteria [6]:

1. Timing (peripartum; last month of pregnancy to 5 months postpartum)
2. Decreased ejection fraction (< 45%)
3. No pre-existing heart disease
4. No other identifiable cause of heart failure

Laboratory Studies

No single laboratory test is diagnostic of PPCM. However, review of laboratory studies may reveal a pattern to help delineate from other differential diagnoses.

A B-type natriuretic peptide (BNP) and troponin may be elevated, suggesting congestive heart disease and cardiac strain.

Complete blood count (CBC), liver function tests (LFTs), lactate dehydrogenase (LDH), uric acid, and fibrinogen will help evaluate for preeclampsia and HELLP

(Hemolysis, Elevated Liver enzymes, Low Platelets) syndrome. An elevated white blood count (WBC) could suggest infectious cardiomyopathy. Elevated aminotransferases (AST > 150 units/L and ALT >100 units/L), thrombocytopenia (platelets $<150 \times 10^9$/L), anemia, decreased fibrinogen, and elevated LDH (> 600 IU/L) will typically diagnose HELLP.

Coagulation markers (PT/PTT/INR) may be helpful for risk stratification because of the increased risk of thromboembolic events. In addition, elevated PTT and PT could suggest HELLP syndrome and/or preeclampsia.

Imaging Findings

Chest radiograph (CXR) will often demonstrate an enlarged cardiac silhouette and pulmonary congestion with vessel cephalization and/or Kerley B lines.

Echocardiogram is the most useful testing modality for diagnosis of PPCM. It will show depressed left ventricular function (< 45%). There will often be right ventricle, left ventricle, or even atrial enlargement but the chambers could also be within the normal size ranges. Valvular function at the mitral and tricuspid may have some regurgitation, but in general, valvular function will be intact. Signs of pulmonary hypertension are possible. Isolated diastolic disfunction may be more suggestive of severe preeclampsia.

Electrocardiogram (ECG) findings are often nonspecific, though sinus tachycardia is the most common finding. There may be nonspecific T-wave or ST segment findings, or the ECG may mirror the findings on the echocardiogram (i.e., atrial enlargement, ventricular hypertrophy).

Diagnosis of PPCM can be confirmed by cardiac catheterization, which will evaluate for wedge pressures and rule out ischemic causes of cardiomyopathy as well as differentiate cardiomyopathy from preeclampsia [7].

Management

The most important emergency interventions should be regarding respiratory and circulatory support. Noninvasive positive pressure ventilation will decrease preload and afterload. Similarly, intubation may be an indicated option. However, third-trimester pregnant patients have a higher risk of becoming hypoxic or apneic during rapid sequence intubation, due to low functional residual capacity and increased basal oxygen metabolic rate.

Circulatory support focuses on optimal intravascular volume and perfusion while maintaining blood flow to the placenta for the gravid patient. The relative decreased volume status of the mother due to decompensated heart failure can compromise uterine perfusion. Administering large volumes of intravenous fluids should be avoided if hypotension or clinical signs of poor perfusion are present. It is critically important to maintain cardiac output using vasopressors or inotropes as needed, though there is no consensus on the best agent to use to promote appropriate circulation in both the mother and the fetus in a case of decompensated PPCM. Consideration should be given to the concept that phenylephrine and norepinephrine, which have more α-agonist receptor activity, may have the potential to cause vasoconstriction of the uterine arteries which could cause placental insufficiency.

Though the patient may be hypertensive, angiotensin converting enzyme (ACE) inhibitors and angiotensin receptor blockers (ARBs) should not be given to pregnant or breastfeeding patients because of possible irreversible renal injury to the fetus or newborn. Diuretics (hydrochlorothiazide, furosemide) may help decrease preload and are safe in pregnancy and with breastfeeding. Hydralazine may help decrease afterload but should only be used postpartum, and it is contraindicated in the gravid patient. Nitrates are useful to decrease both preload and afterload. They are safe during pregnancy but safety during breastfeeding is uncertain.

Thromboembolic prophylaxis is an important consideration due to the hypercoagulable state being intrinsically elevated in the peripartum period. Anticoagulation is indicated when ejection fraction <30% and within 2–3 months following delivery [8]. Heparin and low molecular weight heparin are satisfactory for use during pregnancy or breastfeeding. Warfarin and direct-acting oral anticoagulants (DOACs) should not be used during pregnancy due to possible harm to the fetus.

Specifically, prepartum early fetal heart monitoring should be performed. In the emergency department, bedside duplex ultrasound or Doppler auscultation can obtain a single fetal heart rate. However, continuous fetal heart rate monitoring is usually performed in conjunction with obstetric consultants.

Consultation Considerations

The obstetrics team should be consulted early for fetal heart monitoring and for evaluation for possible emergency cesarean delivery to ensure the best outcome for the mother and the fetus. Prolonged medical therapies for PPCM have the potential to be dangerous for the fetus.

A cardiologist can be consulted for management of cardiogenic shock or decompensated heart failure. In addition, a cardiology consultant can evaluate the patient for cardiac assist devices (e.g., left ventricular assist device (LVAD), extracorporeal membrane oxygenation (ECMO), intra-aortic balloon pump, or cardiac defibrillator).

Cardiology consultants or critical care consultants may continue cardiopulmonary monitoring in an intensive care or other capable unit.

Emergency Department Course and Outcome

The patient was urgently placed on respiratory support using bi-level positive pressure. Her blood pressure dropped to 75/55 mmHg, though her work of breathing significantly improved. She was started on an intravenous continuous epinephrine infusion resulting in improvement of her mean arterial blood pressure and was given an intravenous push of furosemide. The physician performed a point-of-care ultrasound of the heart and the inferior vena cava (IVC), discovering a significantly decreased ejection fraction, no pericardial effusion, grossly normal valvular function, and a plethoric IVC. The physician also identified an intrauterine pregnancy with a fetal heart rate of about 160 beats per minute.

The physician consulted obstetrics emergently for continuous fetal monitoring. She was also given a dose of betamethasone due to the fetus's gestational age. The patient was admitted to an intensive care unit (ICU) where she was emergently evaluated by a heart failure specialist. She received a formal echocardiogram which revealed an ejection fraction of 30%. There were also several episodes of non-sustained ventricular tachycardia captured on the mother's cardiac rhythm monitor.

A few hours later, she complained of abdominal pain and the fetal monitoring was concerning for late decelerations. The patient was taken to the operating room for a stat cesarean section with the obstetrics team and intubated by an obstetric anesthesiologist. The baby required minimal resuscitation (i.e., bag valve mask) and was admitted to the neonatal intensive care unit where she ultimately progressed well.

The mother remained in the ICU for several days and was eventually able to be weaned from vasopressors. She underwent a cardiac catheterization which did not show coronary artery disease, but rather suggested cardiomyopathy. She was evaluated by an electrophysiologist due to the episodes of ventricular tachycardia captured on telemetry during her admission. The hypothesis is that her presentation to the ED may have been syncope due to a non-sustained ventricular arrhythmia caused by her PPCM. Therefore, the patient received an implantable cardiac defibrillator before being discharged from the hospital after a prolonged inpatient stay.

Key Points

- Peripartum cardiomyopathy can present with hypertension, hypotension, or normal blood pressure.
- Cardiac imaging, particularly by point-of-care ultrasound, plays a fundamental role in timely identification of a decreased ejection fracture suggestive of peripartum cardiomyopathy.
- Vasopressor support is an important early intervention that is often necessary when there are signs of cardiogenic shock. However, the potential for compromised placental perfusion can hasten the need for delivery for fetal safety.

References

1. Pearson GD, Veille J-C, Rahimtoola S, et al. Peripartum cardiomyopathy. JAMA. 2000;283(9):1183. https://doi.org/10.1001/jama.283.9.1183.
2. Sliwa K, Hilfiker-Kleiner D, Petrie MC, et al. Current state of knowledge on aetiology, diagnosis, management, and therapy of Peripartum cardiomyopathy (PPCM): a position statement from the heart failure Association of the European Society of cardiology working group on peripartum cardiomyopathy. Eur J Heart Fail. 2010;12(8):767–78. https://doi.org/10.1093/eurjhf/hfq120.

3. Azibani F, Sliwa K. Peripartum cardiomyopathy (PPCM): an update. Curr Heart Fail Rep. 2018;15(5):297–306. https://doi.org/10.1007/s11897-018-0404-x.
4. Patten IS, Rana S, Shahul S, et al. Cardiac angiogenic imbalance leads to peripartum cardiomyopathy. Nature. 2012;485(7398):333–8. Published 2012 May 9. https://doi.org/10.1038/nature11040.
5. Gentry MB, Dias JK, Luis A, Patel R, Thornton J, Reed GL. African-American women have a higher risk for developing peripartum cardiomyopathy. J Am Coll Cardiol. 2010;55(7):654–9. https://doi.org/10.1016/j.jacc.2009.09.043.
6. Elkayam U, Akhter MW, Singh H, et al. Pregnancy-associated cardiomyopathy: clinical characteristics and a comparison between early and late presentation. Circulation. 2005;111(16):2050–5. https://doi.org/10.1161/01.CIR.0000162478.36652.7E.
7. Kealey A. Coronary artery disease and myocardial infarction in pregnancy: a review of epidemiology, diagnosis, and medical and surgical management. Can J Cardiol. 2010;26(6):185–9. https://doi.org/10.1016/s0828-282x(10)70397-4.
8. Arany Z, Elkayam U. Peripartum cardiomyopathy. Circulation. 2016;133(14):1397–409. https://doi.org/10.1161/CIRCULATIONAHA.115.020491.

Evaluating a Newborn

Happy Birthday to You!

Asha Morrow

Case

A newborn girl, less than one minute old, born at 37 weeks and 6 days presents to the emergency department (ED) after her mother precipitously delivered. The family was in the ED having the newborn's older sibling assessed for upper respiratory symptoms when the mother happened to go into active labor. The patient's mother is a 28-year-old (G3P3) who had been having contractions throughout the day. Her water broke while she was sitting at the other child's bedside. Thinking she had more time, the mother remained in the room managing her breathing and the contractions. Eventually, the mother felt the baby crowning and pressed the emergency assist button in the patient room. Upon entering the room, the responding staff found the mother holding the crying newborn with the umbilical cord still attached and the other child sitting patiently in the chair.

- Past medical history: Mother received routine prenatal care starting at 8 weeks; normal anatomy ultrasound at 20 weeks
- Medications: None
- Allergies: No known drug allergies
- Family history: Mother reports Group B Streptococcus screen negative; sexually transmitted infection screen negative; rhesus (Rh) factor positive
- Social history: Household consists of 2 parents and 2 healthy older siblings; mother denies any drug or alcohol use, and she stopped smoking 6 years ago.

A. Morrow (✉)
Department of Pediatrics, Baylor College of Medicine/Texas Children's Hospital, Houston, TX, USA
e-mail: amorrow@bcm.edu

© The Author(s), under exclusive license to Springer Nature Switzerland AG 2024
A. A. Kosoko (ed.), *Emergency Medicine Case-Based Guide*,
https://doi.org/10.1007/978-3-031-70118-4_18

Table 18.1 Point-of-care glucose

Point-of-care glucose	70 mg/dL

Physical Exam

- Vital signs
  - Heart rate: 150 beats/minute
  - Respiratory rate: 46 breaths/minute
  - Temperature: 99.1 °F
  - Oxygen saturation: 96% on room air
  - Weight: 6 lb., 13 oz.
- General appearance: Pink, crying, eyes closed
- HEENT
  - Head: Soft, open fontanelle, no swelling
  - Eyes: Open spontaneously, no conjunctival hemorrhages
  - Ears: Regularly set
  - Nose: No discharge
  - Mouth: No teeth or lesions present
- Heart: Regular, rate, and rhythm, no murmurs present, strong umbilical stump pulse
- Lungs: Clear to auscultation bilaterally; no nasal flaring, grunting, or retractions
- Abdominal/GI: Soft abdomen, bowel sounds present, no hepatosplenomegaly, a gelatinous 3-cord umbilical stump with 2 arteries and 1 vein, no oozing or redness
- Genitourinary: Age appropriate, female-appearing genitalia
- Rectal: Patent anus
- Extremities: Full, symmetric range of motion of all extremities
- Back: No sacral dimple
- Neuro: Symmetric Moro reflex present; plantar and palmar reflexes; strong suck
- Skin: Dry, slight cyanotic appearance to hands and feet, no other lesions present

Pertinent Diagnostic Tests (Table 18.1)

Learning Points

Background

A healthy newborn patient may present to the ED due to an out-of-hospital delivery (e.g., home birth, birth *en route*, having been left at a safe haven, brought from a birthing center). Babies can also unexpectedly be born in the ED itself. A precipitous birth is described as labor lasting less than three hours. Fortunately, precipitous deliveries are rare (about 3% of deliveries in the United States [1]) and generally proceed without significant complications. The births are typically associated with triggers such as chorioamnionitis, hypertension, drug use, or trauma. Presentation to the ED may be associated with mothers who may be critically ill, may not have received prenatal care, may not understand the medical system, lack access to services, may have been in denial or unaware of pregnancy, or simply had a precipitous delivery.

Every baby should receive a postpartum evaluation to determine whether intervention or resuscitation is necessary to optimize the outcome of the newly born child. Understandably, an emergency physician may not have had the experience of seeing a significant number of neonates day-to-day. However, it is important that the physician takes an organized approach to try to identify any areas of concern which may warrant further evaluation. The method of evaluation may vary from provider to provider; however, organization and consistency in evaluation are most important to avoid missing concerning aspects of the history and physical.

Differential Diagnosis Healthy term delivery, transient tachypnea of the newborn, murmur (patent ductus arteriosus, ventricular septal defect, pulmonary branch stenosis) [2], hypoglycemia, sepsis.

History and Physical Exam

The history and the physical exam are the most important factors to consider when determining whether a newborn child is normal or in distress. The history of the child itself is limited to a matter of minutes or hours. However, the mother's history and the prenatal course need to be elicited to determine whether there should be concern for distress in the newborn. If the mother or another representative can provide the information, it is most useful to determine whether the mother has any acute or chronic medical conditions or psychologic conditions. Similarly, if the mother has been on any medications, this should be noted. Prenatal care contributes to optimal outcomes. Whether there was prenatal care and whether there were any abnormal findings, missed components, or variances should be noted. A social history is important because certain social factors can contribute to a higher risk birth compared to an uncomplicated birth, particularly if the mother uses or used any recreational drugs, smoked, or consumed alcohol while pregnant.

The most important historical factor directly related to the child itself is the gestational age. A preterm child is at higher risk for complications. Although things may appear normal on exam, a preterm child would require further observation and investigation. A term delivery is defined at or after 37 weeks.

Regarding physical exams, some important points of consideration differ for newborns versus older children and adults. For most adults and older children, whether imminent resuscitation is indicated by a brief evaluation of the airway, breathing, and circulation. For a newborn, however, a brief general assessment of the child is by evaluation of the tone, color, and respiratory status.

Tone is assessed by evaluating the flexion of the arms and legs. A child with flexed extremities would indicate a good and normal tone. A child with floppy limbs is abnormal and concerning.

If the child is crying, that is very reassuring regarding the respiratory status. It is a simple indicator that the child is breathing effectively and the airway is patent. Though crying can be prompted by minor stimulation (e.g., drying, flicking feet), spontaneous crying is the most reassuring. Of course, one can simply observe the child to see if it is breathing and whether breathing appears labored.

Term infants who have good muscle tone and spontaneous, non-distressed respirations (or a vigorous cry) typically do not require medical intervention [3].

An Apgar score (Table 18.2) is a common and objective measurement summarizing the important items of the general assessment of the newborn and is a means of communicating the health of the newborn. It is often performed at the first minute and again at five minutes of life. Ninety percent of infants with scores ≥ 7 generally do not require intervention [2].

Vital signs of the newborn are very dissimilar from an older child or adult, and they carry different meanings. The most important vital sign on initial evaluation is the heart rate. A normal resting heart rate for a newborn should be 100–180 beats/minute with expectant variability. Anything more or less than this range requires rapid intervention because it could imply that the child is in distress. The heart rate can be counted out by palpation of the umbilical stump, by auscultation of the heart by stethoscope, using a Doppler, by a pulse oximeter, or by a three-lead cardiovascular monitor. Of these options, the most accurate and efficient method is to obtain a measurement from a three-lead monitor. Of note, acrocyanosis (a pink core with blue extremities) is a common and normal finding in a newly born patient. Acrocyanosis typically resolves spontaneously or with warming the child.

Blood pressure is a far less important vital sign for this particular population. Moreover, many facilities are not well-equipped with an appropriately sized neonatal blood pressure cuff. The mean arterial pressure (MAP) typically, at minimum, correlates with the newborn's gestational age (e.g., a 38-week-old infant likely will have a MAP ≥ 38 mmHg); lower values are concerning for hypotension [4].

The most important information about breathing and circulation in the neonate is obtained by observing the child and determining the heart rate. A normal respiratory

Table 18.2 Apgar scoring system using respiratory effort, heart rate, muscle tone, reflexes, and skin color

	0	1	2
Appearance (color)	Blue or pale	Acrocyanosis	Pink
Pulse	0 beats/minute	< 100 beats/minute	$\geq$ 100 beats/minute
Grimace (reflex irritability in response to suction)	Absent	Grimace	Grimace and cough or sneeze
Activity (muscle tone)	Limp	Some flexing of arms and legs	Active motion
Respiratory effort	None	Slow and/or irregular	Regular, strong cry

rate will be 30–60 breaths/minute. Periodic breathing can include pauses of up to 10 seconds and are not associated with respiratory distress. It is important to note that oxygen saturation in a newly born child is interpreted quite differently than other patient populations because the child usually has not yet adapted from a fetal circulatory system. Therefore, it may take about 15 minutes after birth for a newborn to exhibit what most practitioners would consider "normal" oxygen saturation measurements (Table 18.3). If oxygen saturation is obtained, it should be measured as a pre-ductal measurement. This means that the measurement is usually taken from the right hand or wrist before the blood is allowed to mix due to a patent ductus arteriosus. Outside of these parameters, a measurement of oxygen saturation alone should not suffice to initiate supplemental oxygen.

Temperature should be measured for each newborn. Normothermia is described as between 36.5 °C (97.7 °F) and 38 °C (100.4 °F) Neonates may often present with hypothermia rather than fever as a sign of sepsis. Rectal temperatures are typically used to obtain core temperature. If concerned for safety of a rectal temperature, an axillary temperature should be obtained as an alternative [5].

Laboratory Studies

Laboratory studies are generally not indicated in the postpartum period to determine whether a child is sick when a child has an otherwise reassuring history and physical exam. The most useful laboratory test is a point-of-care (POC) glucose. A POC glucose is indicated for asymptomatic newborns who are <37 weeks gestational age, large or small for gestational age, infants of diabetic mothers, and those whose family history predisposes to hypoglycemia (e.g., Beckwith–Wiedemann syndrome) [3]. A POC glucose ≥50 mg/dL in the first 2 hours is considered normal in the asymptomatic neonate [6].

Management

A key element of caring for a precipitously born child in the emergency setting is preparation. Every emergency department should contain supplies specifically set aside for the event of a precipitous birth including an umbilical clamp, scissors, bulb syringe, and clean, dry towels [7]. If unavailable, hemostats can be used as an umbilical clamp and should be placed 2–3 centimeters from the baby's abdomen

Table 18.3 Estimated anticipated pre-ductal oxygen saturation measurements for a newborn minutes after birth

Minutes	Pre-ductal
3	84
4	87
5	92
10	96
15	98

[8]; silk suture can also be used for hemostasis at the umbilicus. If sterile scissors

are not available, a surgical blade can be used. Ideally completed within 30 seconds of birth, a crying term newborn should be dried and warmed; additional stimulation via vigorous rubbing with a towel can be done until the baby cries. These steps often occur simultaneously as the cord is clamped when multiple providers are present [9]. No airway suctioning is needed if there is no concern for airway obstruction or respiratory depression. If the infant is term with good muscle tone and breathing spontaneously, generally the patient does not require imminent intervention and can remain with its mother for skin-to-skin contact and feeding, with only observation and reactionary intervention as indicated thereafter.

Generally healthy term newborns and uncomplicated maternal conditions are admitted to units which can accommodate both the mother and newborn for coordinated routine care and monitoring (e.g., mother/baby unit).

Consultation Considerations

If there is a neonatologist or neonatal delivery/resuscitation team available, it should be activated as soon as delivery is imminent or has occurred, to help manage the newborn with their expertise.

An obstetrician should be consulted if available to manage the mother and her postpartum state.

If physician specialists themselves are not available, nurses or midwives with experience in neonatal management or labor and delivery management may be useful to the emergency care of a precipitous delivery.

Emergency Department Course and Outcome

The newborn was brought into the resuscitation room where her umbilical cord was clamped and cut expeditiously. On examination, it was a normal cord. The crying infant was dried with a towel and then wrapped in a dry blanket to keep her warm. She remained active and with a good tone so was handed over to her mother for skin-to-skin contact and interaction. Her 5-minute Apgar score was 9. Her mother attempted breast feeding, and the child successfully latched and suckled waiting for transfer to the mother/baby unit.

There, the child received a full head-to-toe newborn exam and her newborn screening labs from the pediatric specialist. She continued to feed well and had a bowel movement, passing meconium within 24 hours. She never required phototherapy. Her mother also was demonstrating normal recovery from the delivery process. The child received erythromycin ophthalmic ointment to prevent ophthalmia neonatorum, along with intramuscular vitamin K and hepatitis B vaccination. Her screening for hypoxic congenital heart disease (i.e., pulse oximetry measured at both right hand and foot) [5] was also performed the next day after 24 hours of life and was normal. The child was discharged home on hospital day 2 with her mother and father, who brought a regulation car seat for safe transport.

Key Points

- The primary tenets for determining a normal neonate upon initial evaluation are *term* (gestational age), *tone*, and *tune* (crying and respiratory status).
- The most important initial interventions for a neonate are to dry, warm, and stimulate.
- Routine labs are often not required in term, active neonates. A point-of-care glucose may be necessary for infants with unclear history or risk factors for hypoglycemia.
- A term and otherwise healthy neonate should be admitted to a mother/baby unit for monitoring and routine care.

References

1. Martin JA, Hamilton BE, Osterman MJ, Driscoll AK, Mathews TJ. Births: final data for 2015. Natl Vital Stat Rep. 2017;66(1):1.
2. Gannon C, McKee-Garret T. Newborn Care. In: Guidelines for acute care of the neonate. 30th ed. Houston: Baylor College of Medicine Section of Neonatology, Department of Pediatrics; 2022. p. 184.
3. McKee-Garret T. Overview of the routine management of the healthy newborn infant. In: Post, TW, editor. UpToDate. Waltham: UpToDate; 2022.
4. Batton B. Neonatal Blood Pressure Standards: What is "Normal?" Clin Perinatol. 2020; 47(3):469–485. https://doi.org/10.1016/j.clp.2020.05.008. Pub 2020 May 22.
5. Andescavage NN, Berkowitz D, Soghier L. Neonatal emergencies. In: Fleisher & Ludwig's textbook of pediatric emergency medicine. 7th ed. Philadelphia: Wolters Kluwer; 2016.
6. Dina D, Gannon C. Endocrinology. In: Guidelines for acute care of the neonate. 30th ed. Houston: Baylor College of Medicine Section of Neonatology, Department of Pediatrics; 2022. p. 46.
7. American Academy of Pediatrics, Committee on Pediatric Emergency Medicine, American College of Emergency Physicians, Pediatric Committee, Emergency Nurses Association Pediatric Committee. Joint policy statement—guidelines for care of children in the emergency department. Pediatrics. 2009;124(4):1233–43. https://doi.org/10.1542/peds.2009-1807.
8. Vora S, Dobiesz VA. Emergency childbirth. In: Roberts and hedges' clinical procedure in emergency medicine and acute care. Philadelphia: Elsevier; 2019.
9. Weiner GM, Zaichkin J. Textbook of neonatal resuscitation. 7th ed. Elk Grove Village: American Academy of Pediatrics; 2016.

Neonatal Resuscitation

Let's All Take a Deep Breath

Juliana Jaramillo

Case

Emergency medical services (EMS) responded to a call for a 24-year-old woman in active labor. The woman had not received prenatal care, though she estimates that the fetus is about 8 months gestational age by her last menstrual period. The symptoms started with small volumes of vaginal bleeding last night and have progressed to this morning when she started having severe abdominal pain, contractions and, she believes, leakage of fluids. After arrival to the scene, EMS spent 5 minutes with the mother assessing her and preparing her for transport as she was in labor. A singleton vaginal delivery occurred spontaneously in the ambulance bay upon arrival to the emergency department (ED) after the mother gave one final, large push. The EMS crew clamped and cut the umbilical cord. The baby, however, appeared limp and did not have spontaneous breathing.

- Past medical history: No prenatal care reported. This is the mother's second live birth. The prior delivery was preterm.
- Past surgical history: None
- Medications: None
- Allergies: No known drug allergies
- Social history: Polysubstance abuse (fentanyl, marijuana, and cocaine) periodically through the pregnancy

J. Jaramillo (✉)
Department of Emergency Medicine, East Carolina University Brody School of Medicine, Greenville, NC, USA
e-mail: Jaramilloj21@ecu.edu

   193
A. A. Kosoko (ed.), *Emergency Medicine Case-Based Guide*,
https://doi.org/10.1007/978-3-031-70118-4_19

Physical Exam

- General appearance: Appears small for stated gestational age, not responsive to stimulation
- Heart: Weak brachial pulses with heart rate 40 beats/minute
- Lungs: No spontaneous breathing
- Abdominal/GI: Soft; umbilical cord clear, intact, and clamped
- Neuro: Limp, no spontaneous movement of extremities
- Skin: Pale; cyanotic extremities

Learning Points

Background

When a baby is born, a unique, singular transition occurs, wherein intrauterine physiology converts to extrauterine physiology. Guidelines have been developed, based on best practices, for resuscitation of the newly born baby [1, 2]. These guidelines take into consideration the causes of clinical deterioration and other aspects which differ from resuscitation of an older child or an adult.

Though it may sound daunting, the resuscitation of the newly born child is quite rare. About 10% of babies require some assistance with breathing upon birth, while less than 1% require extensive resuscitative efforts [1, 2].

Resuscitation should begin immediately once a sick neonate is identified by cyanosis, asystole, respiratory distress/arrest, or bradycardia.

However, if a child appears to have a severe congenital malformation or is severely premature, a discussion and introspection should occur regarding the ultimate benefit or futility of resuscitation. Only 9% of children born at 22 weeks gestational age survive to hospital discharge. Resuscitation measures are generally deemed futile prior to 23 weeks [1]. There is limited data to guide when resuscitation efforts should cease, however, after 20 minutes survival rates drop significantly.

Lung development is not complete until approximately 34 weeks' gestation. Prior to 23–24 weeks, the terminal airways of the fetus are not fully developed and typically lack surfactant necessary for proper lung function. The most drastic physiologic change in the baby from intrauterine to extrauterine cardiopulmonary perfusion occurs when the baby takes that first breath, expanding lungs, and causing pulmonary vasodilation for the first time. In utero, blood was being shunted away from the lungs toward the placenta for gas exchange. If a newly born child does require resuscitation, it is generally due to respiratory failure due to a slow-to-adapt or failed cardiopulmonary transition.

Differential Diagnosis hypovolemia from blood loss, maternal intoxicant exposure, meconium aspiration, congenital heart defect, congenital diaphragmatic hernia, hypoglycemia, sepsis.

History and Physical Exam

Inpatient obstetricians and neonatologists often understand that a laboring mother is high risk for a newborn requiring impending resuscitation. However, the emergency setting rarely affords providers the opportunity to know when a newly born child will be presenting to the ED. Therefore, it is rare that an emergency physician will be able to risk-stratify which babies born will require intervention. Most births occurring in the ED are precipitous. Though the resuscitation may commence prior to the opportunity to obtain a history, there are important historical aspects that should eventually be obtained, including the approximate gestational age of the baby, the color of the amniotic fluid leaked, any prenatal complications, and if any prenatal care was obtained. If possible, it may be helpful to know if there were any known risk factors which would increase the likelihood of a resuscitation needing to occur: preeclampsia/eclampsia, maternal substance abuse, no prenatal care, known fetal abnormalities, trauma, placenta previa or abruption, breech birth, and others.

Immediately after birth, a rapid assessment should occur for every baby. This assessment consists of three simple questions:

1. Is the baby of term gestation?
2. Is the baby crying or taking good breaths?
3. Is the muscle tone good?

If the answer to all three of these questions is "yes" or affirmative then, generally, the baby will not require resuscitation and can be handed to the mother or taken to the medical nursery for conservative management (e.g., drying, skin-to-skin, breast feeding, or non-invasive observation).

If any of the questions listed elicits a "no" or negative response, resuscitation should occur in appropriate sequence.

Laboratory Studies

In general, laboratory studies do not have a place in the resuscitation of a critically ill newborn. However, one test which may be helpful in a child who may have demonstrated seizure-like activity or persistent lethargy is a point-of-care glucose to evaluate for hypoglycemia (< 30 mg/dL). Hypoglycemia can be treated with administration of glucose.

Imaging Findings

At the time of resuscitation, imaging studies are generally not indicated. A chest radiograph may be used to confirm endotracheal tube placement or to evaluate for complications of the resuscitation or causes of the cardiopulmonary decline (e.g., pneumothorax, congenital diaphragmatic hernia), but only after the patient has been stabilized.

Management

Minimally Invasive Interventions

The initial steps in stabilizing a newly born child are minimally invasive: warming, clearing the airway when necessary, drying, stimulating the child. Usually, these interventions are performed simultaneously. The body temperature goal for a newborn is 36.5–37.5 °C axillary, and it should be pursued actively for a term birth by utilizing an infant warmer (set to 36.5 °C), a commercial thermal mattress, warm blankets, or by covering a wet newborn in plastic (food- or medical-grade). Hyperthermia and hypothermia are both risky for the newborn and increase rates of complications. Towel drying should be avoided in preterm babies (< 32 weeks' gestation) due to their frail skin and musculoskeletal structures.

Clearing the newly born airway by suctioning should not be performed routinely, as it can induce bradycardia; rather, it should only be done if the child is in respiratory distress or if upper obstructive fluid is visible or audible. Ideally, the mouth should be suctioned prior to the nose to prevent aspiration of fluids in the event the baby is startled upon nasal suctioning. The newborn can also be positioned to assist in keeping the upper airway patent by providing a shoulder roll, chin tilt, jaw thrust, or using an upper airway adjunct such as an oropharyngeal airway or a nasopharyngeal device.

Stimulating the newborn, (e.g., rubbing the child's back, emphatically drying with towels, or flicking the child's feet), may facilitate expansion of the lungs and increase blood flow to the lungs, potentially relieving respiratory distress or apnea.

Monitoring Resuscitation

The greatest guide to success in neonatal resuscitation is the heart rate (HR), which reflects oxygenation and ventilation. The most reliable and least obstructive methods to measure HR are by an SpO2 monitor or a 3-lead cardiac monitor. Umbilical stump palpation is unreliable and difficult to reproduce. Alternatives to measuring the HR include listening with a stethoscope or utilizing a Doppler auscultation to count out HR.

If utilizing an oxygen saturation monitor, it is important to be aware that measurements of oxygen saturations in a newly born child require a different interpretation compared to older children and adults. A HR will be accurate using an oxygen saturation monitor reading at any site on the body, but oxygen saturation itself should be measured in a newly born child before the ductus arteriosus for the most accurate measurement (pre-ductal), which would typically be measured at the right hand or wrist [3]. The percent oxygen saturation of newly born babies should be expected to be in the low 80s in the first 5 minutes of life, not reaching 98–100% until about 15–20 minutes after birth [1, 2].

Oxygen delivery during resuscitation of the newly born child should ideally not be regularly administered at 100% concentration. Unnecessarily administering 100% oxygen can do harm to the neonate and does not necessarily give benefit. Room air should be used for neonatal resuscitation unless an oxygen blender (goal 21–30% fraction of inspired oxygen (FiO2) [2]) is readily available to administer the least amount of supplemental oxygen to obtain the desired response.

A heart rate of more than 100 beats/minute is the goal for a critically ill newborn. When the heart rate drops below 100 beats/minute, urgent intervention (usually respiratory support with positive pressure) is necessary before the HR drops below 60 beats/minute, which would essentially signify cardiovascular distress.

Ventilation

Assisted ventilation should be performed whenever a newborn is in respiratory distress, apneic, or if the HR is <100 beats/minute. Ventilation should be performed at a rate of 40–60 breaths/minute [2] in order to keep the HR > 100 beats/minute.

Ventilation can be augmented by an appropriately sized bag valve mask. However, initiating continuous positive airway pressure (CPAP) by facemask should be considered as an early intervention for newborns who are still breathing spontaneously, even if they are in respiratory distress. CPAP can reduce the need for intubation and mechanical ventilation. Positive end-expiratory pressure (PEEP) can be adjusted as a beneficial respiratory intervention for a newborn.

Many emergency physicians do not have significant experience in endotracheal intubation of a newborn. However, utilizing a laryngeal mask airway (LMA) as a supraglottic device is an equally effective option of providing ventilation. However, LMAs are generally not available for children weighing less than 2000 g or if the child is delivered less than 34 weeks' gestational age.

The decision to place an endotracheal tube may occur if there is meconium visible or for deeper tracheal suctioning, if there is prolonged need for ventilation assistance, or if chest compressions are being performed (Table 19.1).

Chest Compressions and Cardiovascular Support

Most infants in respiratory distress or with HR <100 beats/minute will feedback successful interventions with a normal HR following the specified respiratory interventions. Respiratory intervention is priority and should be optimized before any cardiovascular interventions. If the HR remains below 60 beats/minute after at least 30 seconds of ventilation, chest compressions and administration of drugs should be initiated.

Two-thumb chest compressions (by encircling the baby's chest) are superior to the two-finger technique. The optimal rate is about 120 events/minute (90

Table 19.1 Laryngoscope blade size and endotracheal tube size for the neonate

	Weeks' gestation	Laryngoscope blade size	Endotracheal tube size
Extreme premature	< 28 weeks	00 Miller	2.5
Premature	< 37 weeks	0 Miller	3.0
Term	> 37 weeks	1 Miller	3.5

compressions, 30 breaths), coordinated with ventilation at a ratio of 3:1 (3 chest compressions followed by 1 ventilation). Another way to consider regulating the rate of events is to chant, "One-and-two-and-three-and-bag." An HR check should be performed every 60 seconds.

Epinephrine is only indicated when the HR is persistently <60 beats/minute despite optimal ventilation, oxygenation, and chest compressions lasting more than 60 seconds. The concentration of epinephrine to be used in neonatal resuscitation is 0.1 mg/mL (1 mg / 10 mL) and recommended at a dose of 0.01–0.03 mg/kg (equal to 0.1 to 0.3 mL/kg) to be provided by intravenous (IV) or intraosseous (IO) access every 3–5 minutes. If epinephrine is being administered endotracheally, the concentration is the same, but dosage is slightly higher at 0.05–0.1 mg/kg (0.5–1 mL/kg) [2].

Isotonic crystalloid solution can be administered for persistent bradycardia at 10 mL/kg over 5–10 minutes if the child has experienced suspected blood loss or shows signs of shock. An alternative is type O, Rh-negative packed red blood cells or whole blood.

Epinephrine should be administered through an IV line, or it can be administered by endotracheal tube (less-reliable absorption) if unable to access a peripheral line. Though intraosseous (IO) access is popular in older children and adults, IO is not preferred in the newly born baby due to their size and the risk of it easily being dislodged or developing severe complications such as limb ischemia or infection. The preferred next line of access for a newly born child is an umbilical catheter, central venous access (Fig. 19.1).

Umbilical vein catheterization

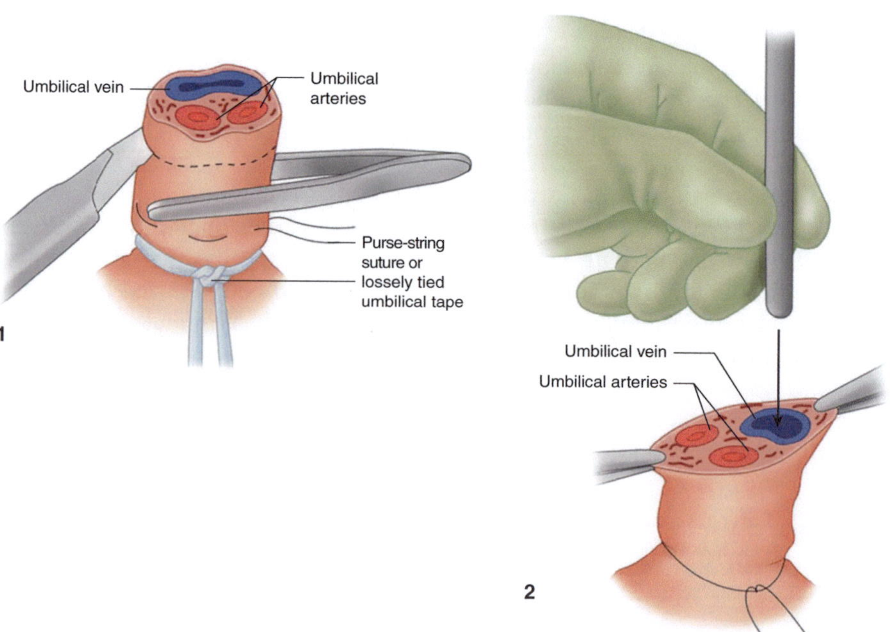

Fig. 19.1 Umbilical vein catheterization technique

Consultation Considerations

For any precipitous birth presenting to the emergency department, a neonatologist or pediatrician should be consulted as soon as possible for management assistance and transfer of care. The child will ultimately need to be admitted to a neonatal intensive care unit.

Emergency Department Course and Outcome

The baby was placed on an infant warmer and on initial evaluation, there was concern that the baby was preterm based on the mother's report and size, but not less than 32 weeks' gestation. The baby was apneic despite efforts to stimulate by drying with warm towels, along with clearing and repositioning of the airway.

The emergency team immediately began communications to identify a receiving neonatal intensive care unit as they began resuscitative efforts. Nursing connected the child to a heart rate monitor, temperature sensor, and a pulse oximeter. The baby was found to be bradycardic with a HR of 48 beats/minute. Despite 60 seconds of minimally invasive measures, the baby remained limp and bradycardic. The resuscitation team initiated positive pressure ventilation (PPV) with an infant bag valve mask with room air. Despite 30 seconds of PPV, there was no clinical improvement. Using 2-person ventilation, the team checked for an appropriate mask seal, chest rise, and even increased the FiO2 administered. After 30 more seconds of continuous PPV without improvement of the baby's heart rate, the team decided to use endotracheal intubation to optimize ventilation of the baby.

Unfortunately, despite appropriate ventilation, the baby's heart rate remained <60 beats/minute. After 60 seconds of chest compressions and one dose of epinephrine administered by the endotracheal tube, the child's HR was noted to be 110 beats/minute on the monitor. With failed attempts at peripheral IV access and an unsuccessful IO attempt, an umbilical vein catheter was placed using sterile technique. An epinephrine infusion was started through the umbilical vein.

The patient was sent by flight with a neonatal transport team for admission and continued workup and management in the neonatal intensive care unit.

Key Points

- Not all newborns require routine suctioning, but if the baby is in respiratory distress, suction the mouth then the nose.
- Early and proper ventilation is usually the most critical and effective intervention in neonatal resuscitation.
- Heart rate is the greatest indicator of newborn distress and should guide progress of resuscitation.

- Consider early continuous positive airway pressure (CPAP) for a child in respiratory distress or placing a laryngeal mask airway (LMA) device instead of early endotracheal intubation.
- Neonatal resuscitation should primarily be performed with room air or blended oxygen rather than 100% oxygen which can do harm and does not give mortality benefit.

References

1. Myers SR, Schinasi DA, Nadel FM. Cardiopulmonary resuscitation. In: Shaw KN, Fleisher GR, Ludwig S, editors. Fleisher & Ludwig's textbook of pediatric emergency medicine. 7th ed. Philadelphia: Wolters Kluwer; 2021. p. 40–51.
2. Weiner GM, Zaichkin J, editors. Textbook of neonatal resuscitation. 8th ed. Itasca: American Academy of Pediatrics; 2021.
3. Dawson JA, Kamlin CO, Wong C, te Pas AB, O'Donnell CP, Donath SM, Davis PG, Morley CJ. Oxygen saturation and heart rate during delivery room resuscitation of infants <30 weeks' gestation with air or 100% oxygen. Arch Dis Child Fetal Neonatal Ed. 2009;94(2):F87–91. https://doi.org/10.1136/adc.2008.141341.

Appendix: Emergency Ultrasound and the Pregnant Patient

Carrie Bakunas and Rachel C. Bower

Point-of-Care Ultrasound

Point-of-care ultrasound (POCUS) is important in evaluation of pregnant patients because it provides real-time bedside visualization of the fetus, uterus, and other pelvic structures. This allows for early detection of potential issues, such as miscarriage, ectopic pregnancy, and fetal distress. Early diagnosis facilitates prompt intervention and better patient outcomes. The portability and accessibility of modern ultrasound machines make them a valuable tool in both low- and high-resource settings.

The use of POCUS enables the clinician to perform the ultrasound in real time at the patient's bedside. These real-time images can immediately be correlated with the patient's symptoms, and any changes in a critical patient's condition can be more rapidly detected and intervened upon. POCUS should be considered a routine extension of practice in caring for pregnant patients. It can provide immediate answers in potentially life-threatening situations. Furthermore, because of its timeliness, it has the added benefit of shortening the length of stay for pregnant patients presenting to the emergency department.

POCUS is different from a conventional radiology-performed ultrasound in that it is a rapid and limited study performed at the bedside for a specific diagnostic or therapeutic purpose. The ultrasound is typically performed by the same clinician treating the patient, providing the additional advantage of knowing a patient's history and symptoms during interpretation of the ultrasound. POCUS, however, is not a substitute for an in-depth prenatal or diagnostic ultrasound scan, and it does not obviate the need for comprehensive sonography during pregnancy. It is important for the clinician to understand the limitations of point-of-care ultrasound. POCUS is invaluably useful in answering pertinent clinical questions but does not reflect the entirety of pathologies that can affect pregnant women or their fetuses. If POCUS

C. Bakunas · R. C. Bower
Department of Emergency Medicine, McGovern School of Medicine, University of Texas Health Sciences Center at Houston, Houston, TX, USA

A. A. Kosoko (ed.), *Emergency Medicine Case-Based Guide*,
https://doi.org/10.1007/978-3-031-70118-4

provides unexpected or indeterminate findings, patients should be sent for comprehensive sonography.

Modern obstetrical care relies heavily on the use of ultrasound. While there remains a role for comprehensive imaging, POCUS enhances emergency patient care of pregnant patients by facilitating interpretation of ultrasound findings rapidly and within a dynamic clinical context at the patient's bedside.

Obstetric Point-of-Care Ultrasound Basics

The use of POCUS should be an extension of the clinician's evaluation of a pregnant patient. Specific indications for emergency ultrasound in pregnancy include abdominal or pelvic pain, vaginal bleeding, or maternal trauma. The majority of obstetric ultrasounds can be completed using a 2–5 MHz curvilinear probe for transabdominal views. The ultrasound machine should be set to the "obstetric" preset so that appropriate calculations and measurements are available. The name of this preset will vary based upon the machine being used, and there may even be trimester-specific options. There are several general tips to help facilitate image acquisition. The examiner should place the focal point in the center of the screen and should adjust the depth and gain accordingly. Additionally, one must use an adequate amount of transducer gel. When the patient has a full bladder, it provides easier visualization uterus and adnexa by pushing the uterus superiorly, out of the pelvis, providing clearer pictures.

Patient positioning is important for all ultrasound studies. The patient should be in a supine position and comfortable with legs extended on the bed. Also, as with all ultrasounds, one must scan the structure of interest in two planes. When scanning the uterus, one should scan in both the sagittal and transverse planes. In the sagittal plane, the probe indicator should point toward the patient's head. For the transverse view, the probe indicator should point toward the patient's right side.

Ectopic Pregnancy

Transabdominal transverse and longitudinal views of a left adnexal ectopic pregnancy (Fig. 2.2). Within the uterus itself, there is no discernible gestational sac, but rather a heterogenous mass with complex fluid likely representing hemorrhage and clot. In the left adnexa, there is a complex mass with a hyperechoic ring without definitive gestational sac or fetal pole and a small stripe of surrounding free fluid. In the right upper quadrant view, note the anechoic strip of fluid seen in Morrison's pouch (hepatorenal space) indicating free fluid present in the abdomen.

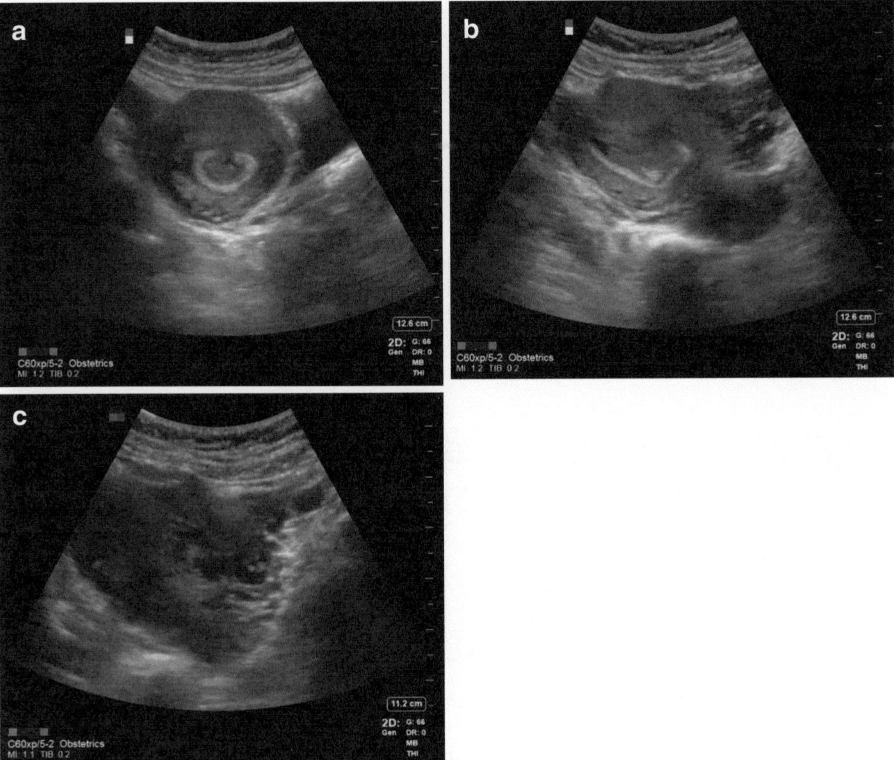

Fig. 2.2 Point-of-Care Pelvic Ultrasound, (**a**) Long uterus view, (**b**) Short uterus view, (**c**) Adnexa: No intrauterine pregnancy identified in uterus, abnormal adnexa. (Images courtesy of C. Bakunas, MD and R. Bower)

Molar Pregnancy

Transabdominal transverse and longitudinal views of a molar pregnancy reveals an enlarged uterus with complex, heterogenous material within the endometrium with a few scattered irregular, hypoechoic cystic spaces. These cystic areas give rise to the classic "snowstorm" or "bunch of grapes" appearance (Figs. 3.3 and 3.6).

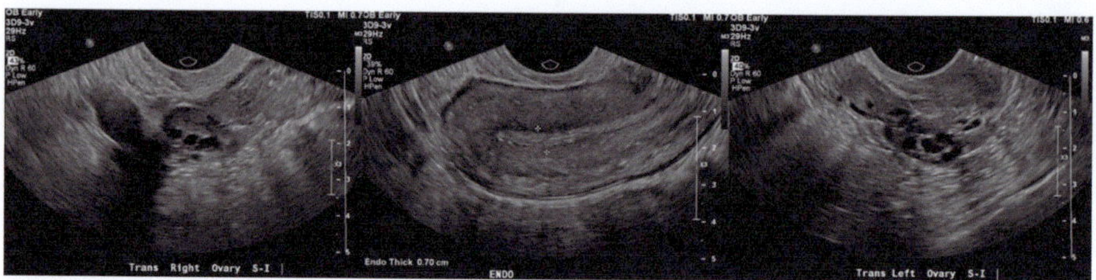

Fig. 3.3 Point-of-Care Pelvic Ultrasound: 8.9 × 4.3 × 5.8 cm slightly heterogenous uterus with cervical fibroid measuring 2.1 × 1.5 × 2.4 cm. Endometrial thickness 0.7 cm with no in-trauterine gestational sac, no definitive molar pregnancy. No adnexal abnormality or enlarged theca lutein cysts. Bilateral normal-appearing ovaries with follicles. (O. Clement's own image)

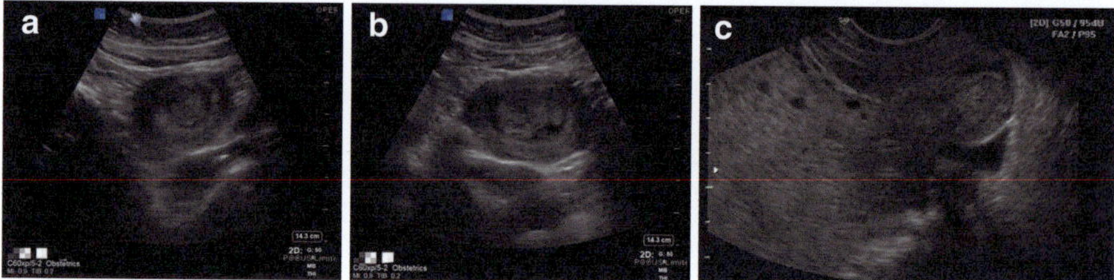

Fig. 3.6 Pelvic Ultrasound (**a**) Long uterus view (**b**) Short uterus view, (**c**) Transvaginal view: Enlarged uterus without a definitive intrauterine pregnancy. Abnormal appearing intrauterine contents. (Images courtesy of C. Bakunas, MD and R. Bower, MD)

Spontaneous Abortion

A threatened abortion is defined as vaginal bleeding that occurs during pregnancy, whereas an incomplete abortion is characterized by some, but not all, of the products of conception passing. This ultrasound shows a confirmed intrauterine pregnancy (Fig. 4.1). A fetal heart rate must be identified to determine whether it is a live, viable pregnancy (threatened abortion) versus a pregnancy which is not viable (missed abortion). Fetal bradycardia or a large subchorionic hemorrhage (> 2/3 the gestational sac) could suggest a poor fetal outcome.

An inevitable or incomplete abortion is seen on transverse and longitudinal transabdominal ultrasound (Fig. 4.3). There is heterogeneous material and complex fluid within the uterus, likely representing hemorrhage and products of conception. Note the irregularly shaped gestational sac without any discernible yolk sac or fetal pole within the vaginal vault, best seen on the longitudinal view. An evaluation of the patient's cervix will determine the diagnosis. Serial bedside or formal ultrasounds can be performed as the tissue passes from the lower segment of the uterus through the endocervical canal into the vaginal vault.

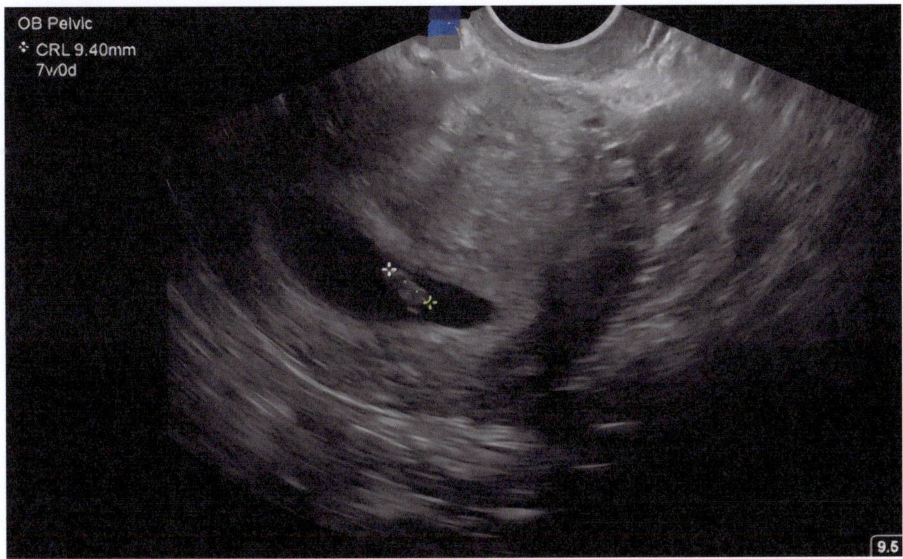

Fig. 4.1 Point-of-care pelvic ultrasound (POCUS): Live intrauterine pregnancy with fetal heart rate of 150 beats/minute. Estimated age by crown rump length is 7 weeks and 0 days. (Image courtesy of Carrie Bakunas, MD.)

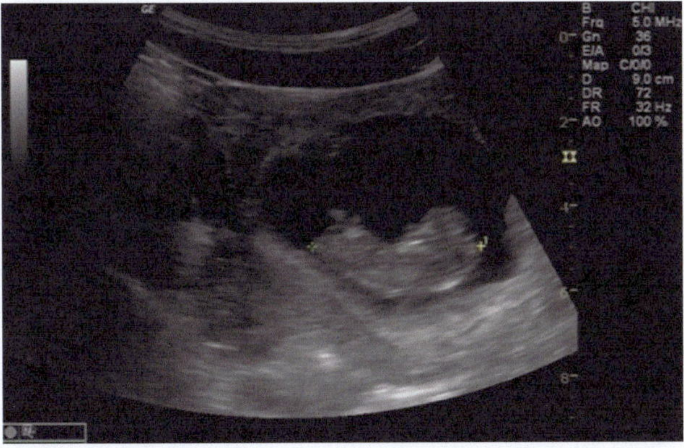

Fig. 4.3 Transabdominal Pelvic Ultrasound: Normal intrauterine pregnancy. (Images courtesy of C. Bakunas, MD and R. Bower, MD)

First Trimester Uterine POCUS

Transabdominal view of an early intrauterine pregnancy at roughly 10 weeks is provided (Fig. 4.4). M-mode, which provides a visual representation of motion over time along the cursor, is used to measure fetal heart rate by placing the curser through the fetal heart and then using the caliper to measure the subsequent sinusoidal wave created by the oscillating heart. Finally, the crown-rump length can be used to date the pregnancy once the embryo is visible by measuring the maximal embryo length (excluding the yolk sac).

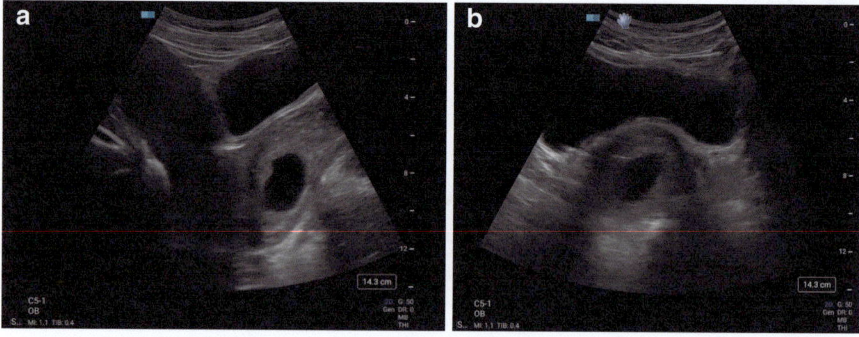

Fig. 4.4 Transabdominal Pelvic Ultrasound (**a**) Long uterus view, (**b**) Short uterus view: No confirmed intrauterine pregnancy. (Images courtesy of C. Bakunas, MD and R. Bower, MD)

Second Trimester Uterine POCUS

Transabdominal, transverse, and longitudinal views of a normal second trimester pregnancy of 20 weeks and 6 days are provided (Figs. 7.2 and 7.3). The placenta is located anteriorly in location (the hyperechoic density seen adhered to the endometrium on the left upper portion of the longitudinal and sagittal images). Femur diaphysis length can be used for pregnancy dating by obtaining a longitudinal view of the femoral shaft and measuring along the ossified portion of the bone. Likewise, biparietal diameter can be used to determine gestational age by measuring from the outer edge of the near calvarial wall to the inner edge of the far wall at the level of the third ventricle and thalamus.

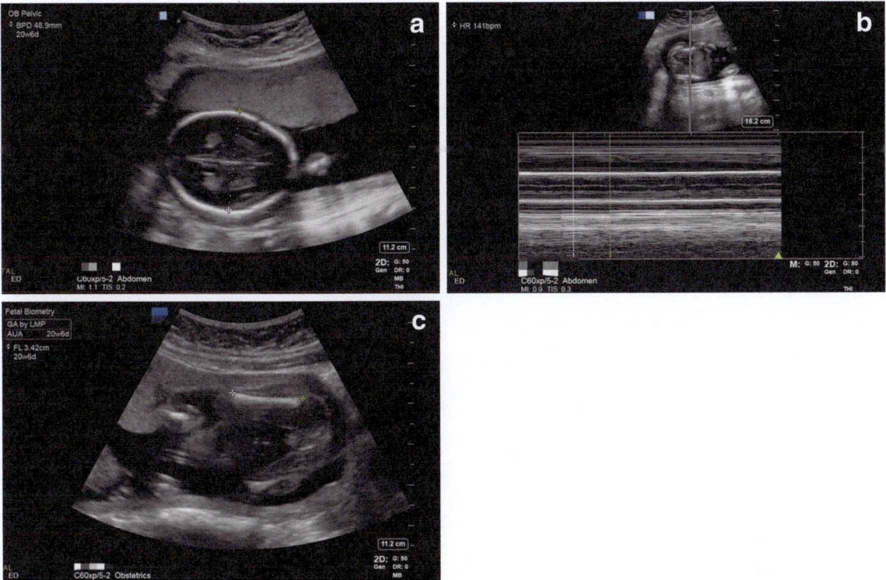

Fig. 7.2 Point-of-care transabdominal ultrasound (**a**) Biparietal diameter, (**b**) Fetal heart rate, (**c**) Femur length: Intrauterine pregnancy at 20 weeks and 6 days and fetal heart rate of 141 beats per minute. (Images courtesy of C. Bakunas and R. Bower)

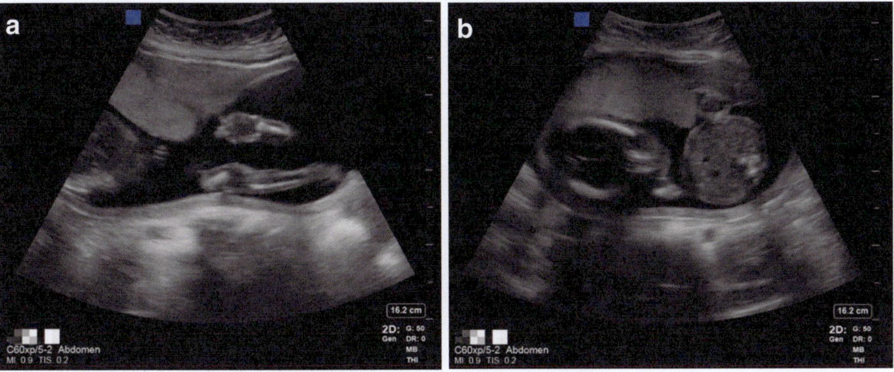

Fig. 7.3 Point-of-Care transabdominal ultrasound (**a**) Long view, (**b**) Short view: Normal intrauterine pregnancy at 20 weeks and 6 days gestational age. (Images courtesy of C. Bakunas, MD and R. Bower, MD)

Thromboembolic Disease

An acute deep vein thrombus typically demonstrates an increased vascular diameter, a noncompressible segment of the vessel, loss of phasic flow or color flow, observed intraluminal material, or lack of augmentation of flow with calf squeeze (Fig. 9.4).

Echocardiogram exam demonstrating findings of a pulmonary embolism with right heart strain and a blood clot in transit (Fig. 9.6). On the parasternal long view, there is a dynamic left ventricle and the enlarged right ventricle. Similarly, in the apical four chamber view, the two ventricles are roughly the same size, indicating right heart enlargement and strain. From the inferior vena cava view, a large, hyperechoic, mobile blood clot extending from the hepatic vein caudally can be seen. The blood clot can again be seen in the subxiphoid view as a hyperechoic, mobile density within the right atrium. In this view, right heart strain is again evident with enlargement compared to the left heart.

Fig. 9.4 Doppler ultrasound right lower extremity (DUS RLE): Inability to completely compress common femoral vein. (Images courtesy of Rachel Bower, MD)

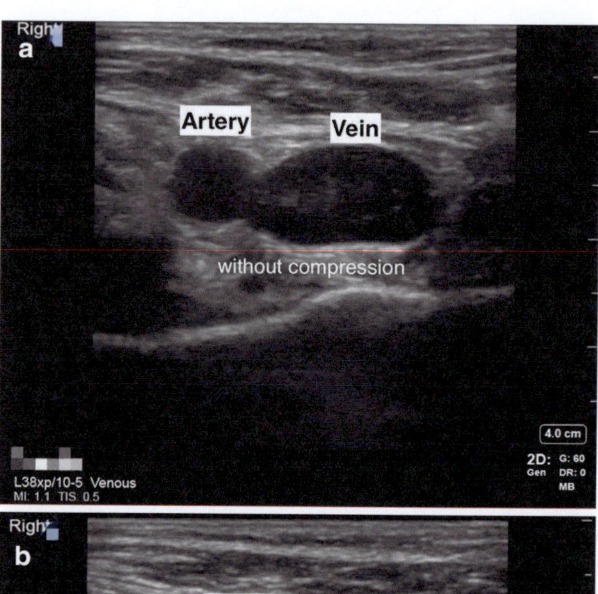

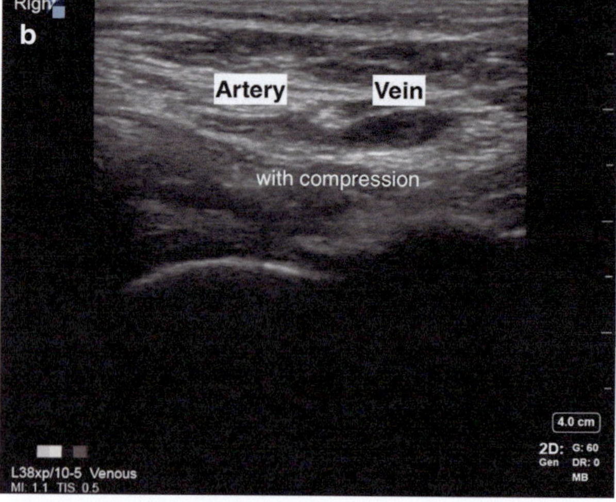

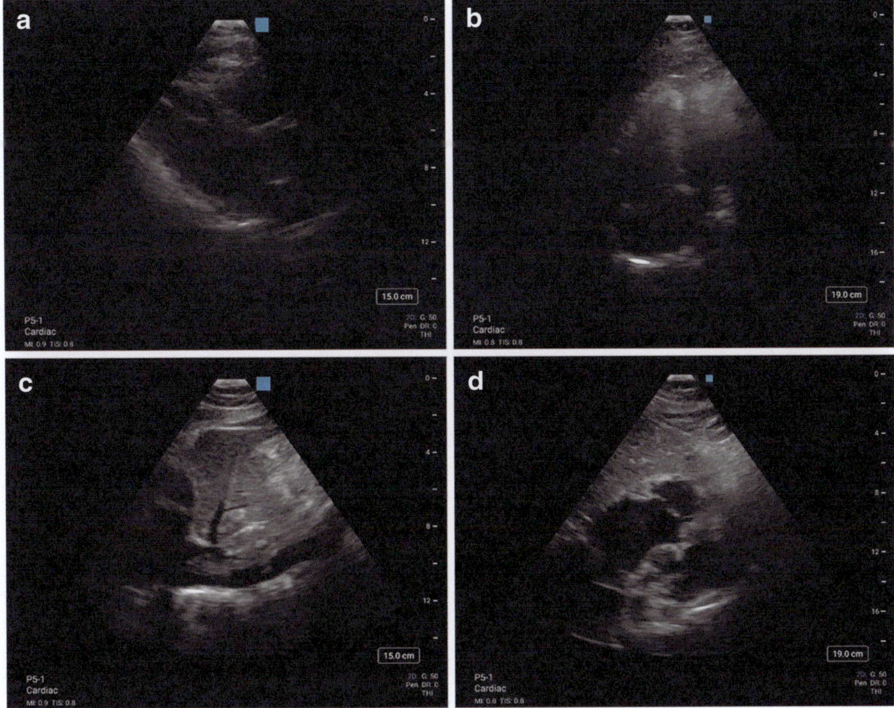

Fig. 9.6 Point-of-Care Cardiac Ultrasound (echocardiogram). (**a**) Parasternal long view, (**b**) Apical four-chamber view, (**c**) Inferior vena cava view, (**d**) Subxiphoid view: Right heart strain and blood clot

Peripartum Cardiomyopathy

Echocardiogram exam demonstrates peripartum cardiomyopathy (Fig. 17.4). On the parasternal long axis, there is left ventricular chamber dilation and globally reduced ejection fraction, qualitatively evidenced by poor inward contraction of the endocardial borders of the left ventricle (less than 50% change in chamber size during systole) and minimal movement of the anterior leaflet of the mitral valve toward to inter ventricular septum. Similarly, the apical four-chamber view demonstrates a globally reduced ejection fraction. The inferior vena cava is dilated with minimal respirophasic variation, indicating high central venous pressure and volume overload with poor forward flow.

Longitudinal images of the bilateral anterior chest wall (Fig. 17.5). Diffuse B-lines, defined as hyperechoic, vertical artifacts originating at the pleural lining and extending deep into the lung parenchyma without attenuation, can be seen while scanning the anterior chest in patients with interstitial edema. Three or more B-lines per intercostal space are considered pathologic. In these images, the pulmonary edema is so severe that it appears as almost complete "white-out" of the intercostal space, as the innumerable B-lines coalesce.

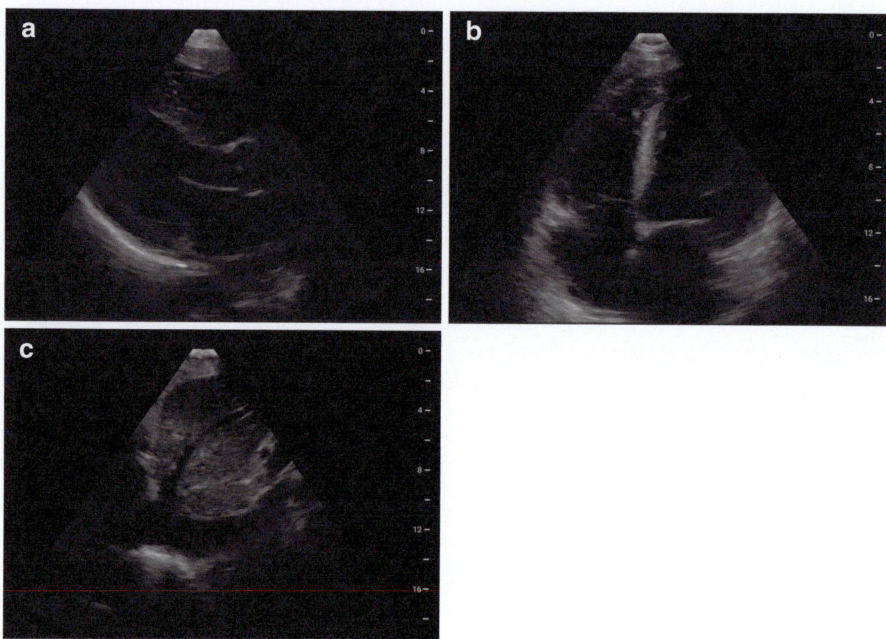

Fig. 17.4 Point-of-care cardiac ultrasound (echocardiogram) (**a**) Parasternal long axis (**b**) apical four-chamber view (**c**) inferior vena cava view: reduced ejection fraction

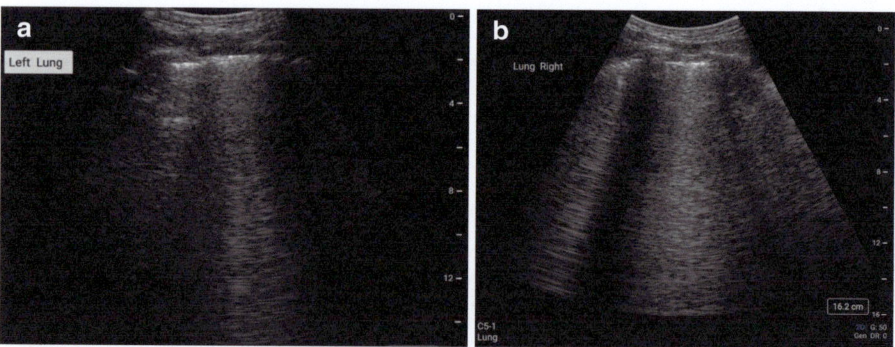

Fig. 17.5 Point-of-care thoracic ultrasound of (**a**) left lung and (**b**) right lung: diffuse B-lines

Index